AF352330

L. F. Hollender · P. Lehnert · M. Wanke

Acute Pancreatitis

Acute Pancreatitis

An Interdisciplinary Synopsis

L. F. Hollender · P. Lehnert · M. Wanke
In collaboration with M. Nagel

Prefaces by
F. Nagao, Tokyo, and G. L. Nardi, Boston

Urban & Schwarzenberg
Munich-Vienna-Baltimore 1983

Authors' addresses:

Professor L. F. Hollender, M.D., Dr.h.c. Dr.h.c., F.A.C.S.
Service de Chirurgie Générale 1 et de Chirurgie Digestive
Centre Hospitalier Universitaire de Strasbourg Hautepierre
Université L. Pasteur
F-67098 Strasbourg Cedex

Priv.-Doz. Dr. med. Peter Lehnert
Medizinische Klinik Innenstadt der Universität München

Prof. Dr. med. Michael Wanke
Chief Physician, Pathological Institute
Kreiskrankenhaus Rendsburg
Akademisches Lehrkrankenhaus für die Universität Kiel

Prof. Dr. med. Martin Nagel
Formerly Chief Physician, General Surgery,
Krankenhaus Ludwigsburg
Akademisches Lehrkrankenhaus für die Universität Heidelberg

Fusahiro Nagao, M.D., F.A.C.S.
Professor and Chairman
Second Department of Surgery
Jikei University School of Medicine
Tokyo

George L. Nardi, M.D.
Professor of Surgery, Visiting Surgeon
Harvard Medical School
Massachusetts General Hospital
Boston, Mass.

Library of Congress Cataloging in Publication Data

Hollender, Louis F.:
Acute pancreatitis : an interdisciplinary
synopsis / L. F. Hollender ; P. Lehnert ;
M. Wanke. In collab. with M. Nagel. Pref. by
F. Nagao and G. L. Nardi. – Munich ; Vienna ;
Baltimore : Urban and Schwarzenberg, 1983.
  Dt. Ausg. u.d.T.: Hollender, Louis F.:
Akute Pankreatitis
  ISBN 3-541-70841-7 (Munich)
  ISBN 0-8067-0841-7 (Baltimore)
NE: Lehnert, Peter:; Wanke, Michael:

Registered tradenames (trademarks) are not always specially identified. The lack of such identification should not be taken to mean that such names may be freely used.

All rights, including those of reprinting, reproduction in any form, and translation into other languages are reserved by the authors and publisher. Without written approval of the publisher, duplication of the book or parts thereof by photomechanical means (photocopy, microfiche), or its storage, systematic utilization, or dissemination by use of electronic or mechanical systems, is not permissible (except in such special cases as specifically cited in §§ 53, 54 of the German Copyright Law).
Production: Kastner & Callwey, Munich
© Urban & Schwarzenberg 1983

ISBN 3-541-70841-7 München
ISBN 0-8067-0841-7 Baltimore

Dedicated to his venerable academic teacher, Prof. Dr. med. Dres. h.c. W. Doerr, the founder of the modern pathomorphology of pancreatitis and pioneer in the elucidation of its pathogenesis as the basis for new clinical, diagnostic, and therapeutic insights.

For all authors: *Michael Wanke*
Autumn 1983

Prefaces

The therapy of acute and especially of hemorrhagic-necrotizing pancreatitis frequently includes surgical treatment of its complications; the inherent problems are ever-present and of immediate concern. Proper treatment of these complications presupposes an understanding of the pathophysiology and pathomorphology, as also an awareness of the limited informative value of methods of clinical chemistry, radiological and sonographic examination, and knowledge of the symptomatology and the disease course.

On the basis of such knowledge, the surgeon may also be able to plan an ideal intervention at the ideal time.

The present monograph persuasively demonstrates the authors' eminent experience. It conveys desirable information and will prove extremely valuable to all physicians faced with the need to treat patients who have acute pancreatitis.

Prof. G. L. Nardi, Boston

The treatment of acute and, in particular, hemorrhagic-necrotizing pancreatitis requires exact knowledge founded on practical experience. This is an indispensable prerequisite in this frequently severe disease with its serious diagnostic and therapeutic problems and consequences. Even though there have been numerous publications on this subject in the past, a monograph reflecting current knowledge and experience and providing competent guidelines for management is more than desirable.

For the treatment of acute pancreatitis, the contents of the present monograph represent an important guide to worldwide scientific experience and treatment modalities employed in current clinical practice. The authors have made a wise and serious-minded effort to evaluate and at the same time coordinate the immense wealth of available reported data and experience, and so to lay the basis for proper understanding and, above all, for optimal therapeutic procedures. The monograph will surely prove of great value for this reason and attract worldwide interest.

I know of no other book at this time that offers so excellent a presentation or matches it in practical utility.

Prof. F. Nagao, Tokyo

Foreword

There is no consensus about the definition of acute pancreatitis. The term acute pancreatitis is synonymously applied to different disease forms and functional states of the gland, depending on the particular discipline or study group. This is a hindrance to the interpretation of clinical data and to the assessment of treatment results, especially with respect to the reduction of the mortality rate and the evaluation of side effects.

It has been the purpose of the present monograph to arrive at a uniform definition of this complex disease as well as to describe the current state of knowledge and experience from an interdisciplinary point of view and thus make it more readily accessible. This synopsis is designed to furnish a useful reference work for all colleagues who are involved in the care of patients with acute pancreatitis.

The authors are indebted to the publishers, Urban & Schwarzenberg, Munich, and notably Mr. Bischoff, for their extraordinary cooperation, and to Bayer AG, Leverkusen, for suggesting and supporting this publication.

Munich, September 1983

L. F. Hollender
P. Lehnert
M. Nagel
M. Wanke

Table of Contents

Table of Contents for the Plate Figures

between Page	Plate	Figur	Chapter
34/35	I	4	3
	II	7, 13	4
	III	14, 15	4
	IV	16, 17, 18	4
	V	19	4
	VI	20, 21	4
	VII	22, 23	4
	VIII	25, 26, 27	4
	IX	35, 36, 37, 38	4
	X	39	4
	XI	40	4
	XII	41, 42, 43, 44, 55	4
114/115	XIII	62, 63, 64	10
	XIV	66	11
	XV	67, 68, 69	11
	XVI	70, 71, 72	11

Chapter 1 – Introduction

Acute autodigestive pancreatitis is based on pathomorphological changes and biochemical conditions that cannot be described and defined adequately and precisely in a stereotyped sentence. In view of the generally complex symptomatology and the widely variable manifestations of this disease, we need to consider especially the principal pathogenetic factors and mechanisms. Accordingly, acute pancreatitis may be divided into three large varieties:

1. Biliary pancreatitis
2. Lipolytic pancreatitis
3. Proteolytic pancreatitis

Causing dyschylia, edema, and disturbances of blood flow and circulation, the autodigestive inflammation specific to pancreatitis may lead in severe cases to partial or total necrosis. This in turn gives rise to specific clinical states and to disease courses of varying severity.

The latter range from a mild form of edematous pancreatitis, with or without adipose tissue necrosis, to the extremely serious picture of the classic abdominal drama according to Dieulafoy. This involves partial or subtotal to total glandular necrosis with all the resultant local and general complications which not infrequently end in death. It is the extreme variant of this diagnostically and therapeutically most challenging gastroenterological disease.

Acute pancreatitis is thus an outstanding example of a test for optimal interdisciplinary management.

Chapter 2 – Etiology

The general clinical incidence of acute pancreatitis is less than 1%. A collective survey by Link, based on 398,060 autopsies, revealed an 0.35% incidence of pancreatic necrosis (1397 cases). Wanke, [480] in a study based on 15,697 autopsies, found 172 cases (1.1%) of acute pancreatitis (98 male patients, 74 female patients).

The age group affected most depends largely on the etiology. Alcoholic pancreatitis tends to occur more often in younger men (ages 30–40 years), whereas the biliary form related to gallstone disease is seen in older women (ages 60–70). Wanke reported the age and sex distribution shown in Table 1 for 172 cases of acute pancreatitis. According to Sarles the male to female ratio is 61% to 39%. Today it is generally believed that the two sexes are equally affected, if special note is taken of the fact that the distribution is chiefly dependent on the etiology [290, 401, 402, 480].

Table 1. Age distribution of 172 cases of acute pancreatitis that were found among 15,697 autopsies performed between 1963 and 1981 (Wanke)

Age (years)	Men	Woman
0–10	1	0
11–20	1	0
21–30	4	1
31–40	15	3
41–50	12	3
51–60	23	12
61–70	26	27
over 70	16	28
Total	98	74

2.1 Frequency of etiological factors

The etiological factors of the disease are numerous, complex and often interwoven, varying geographically from one country to another. We shall divide them into three large groups according to the frequency or rarity of their occurrence (Table 2).

Table 2. Frequency of etiological factors in acute pancreatitis

A.   Principal factors
1. Cholecystocholedocholithiasis
2. Alcoholism
3. Abdominal surgery – postoperative pancreatitis
4. Intraoperative endoscopy of biliary and pancreatic ducts
5. Blunt abdominal trauma

Table 2. Continuation

B. Less common factors
    1. Endocrine diseases (polyadenomatosis, hyperparathyroidism, Cushing's disease)
    2. Pregnancy, hyperlipoproteinemia, pancreatitis following use of oral contraceptives
    3. Drugs (corticosteroids, diuretics)
    4. Immunological-allergic factors
    5. Neurogenic pancreatitis
    6. Hereditary pancreatitis
    7. Virally induced pancreatitis
    8. Parasitic pancreatitis

C. Pancreatitis secondary to shock and acidosis
    (see Chapter 4, Pathogenesis and Morphogenesis)

2.2 Cholecystocholedocholithiasis

The combination of cholelithiasis and acute pancreatitis is a frequently encountered phenomenon. According to Goebell, it may even be found to be the cause of approximately 45–51% of all cases of acute pancreatitis. Molander and Bell discovered a gallstone disease in 36% of the men and in 70% of the women among 160 autopsied patients who had died of acute pancreatitis. They compared their figures with Ludlow's autopsy data, which out of 4800 autopsies of individuals who had not suffered from acute pancreatitis. Cholelithiasis was found to be present in 6% of the men and 10% of the woman. The authors draw the conclusion that cholelithiasis occurs 6 times as frequently in patients with acute pancreatitis. Howard noted that 168 of 353 patients with acute pancreatitis (48%) had cholelithiasis at the same time. We ourselves found the interrelation between pancreatitis and cholelithiasis confirmed in 1144 (39%) out of 2914 cases cited in the literature [223].

Compared with cholecystolithiasis, the risk is increased by 15% and in extreme cases to 100% in choledocholithiasis [159, 160, 201, 223, 293, 319].

Leaving aside the special case of a gallstone wedged into the ampulla of Vater (the Opie syndrome), it is nonetheless difficult to explain precisely what pathogenetic role and significance lithiasis actually has. The clinical experience is incontestable: Surgical treatment of cholelithiasis to remove the stone and eliminate the obstruction to outflow can certainly stop recurrent attacks of pancreatitis. Thus, Howard observed episodes of pancreatitis in 53% of 40 patients. Cholelithiasis had been present for more than 4 years. In the same period only 5 out of 160 surgically treated patients (3%) had further attacks of pancreatitis, indicating a transition to the chronically relapsing disease form [223].

The morphological picture and the intrapancreatic distribution pattern of biliary reflux pancreatitis are determined mainly by the variants of duct anatomy with their interrelations between the common bile duct and the major or minor pancreatic duct and by the presence or absence of accessory pancreatic duct openings into the common bile duct (see Chapter 4).

The proximal duct system in the pancreas has a wide range of variability with respect to the topography of its openings. That portion of the duct which generally opens into a common papilla with the distal ductus choledochus is called the major pancreatic duct or duct of Wirsung. In addition, a minor, accessory pancreatic duct (duct of Santorini) can separately open into the duodenum at 2–3 cm proximal to the major pancreatic duct. This orifice, however, unlike the papilla of Vater, lacks a sphincter. In terms of the course and opening topography of the ducts there are a number of variants (Figs. 1a and 1b). The knowledge concerning this duct variability is important clinically, particularly in ulcer operations when duodenal ulcers extending postpylorically toward the pancreas are to be resected. In the exceptional case postoperative pancreatitis is bound to develop if, because of the surgeon's failure to recognize the separate proximal opening or a sole opening via the accessory duct, the outflow of secretions is prevented by ligation, as a result of which the pathogenetically decisive edema predisposing to pancreatitis is brought about.

Thus, the anatomical "fate" is one of the factors that determine whether a pancreatitic process is confined to the head of the pancreas or involves the whole gland. If there is a communication between the major and the minor papilla, the duct of Santorini can function as an overflow valve despite impaction of a calculus in the region of the papilla. In such cases the lodged stone will only cause edema at the head of the pancreas and the full-blown picture of hemorrhagic-necrotizing pancreatitis may never develop (see Chapter 4).

According to Baldwin, [27] common and separate biliary and pancreatic duct openings occur in the following ratio of frequency: in 76 cases that were studied, a common opening of the duct systems was seen 49 times and a separate opening 27 times.

Finally, in the presence of cholelithiasis pancreatitis can develop canalicularly, via small accessory channels in the distal bile duct (inflammation of head of pancreas), when there is an impacted papillary stone (Opie syndrome), or through a non canalicular way by the lymphogenous-hematogenous route as a referred inflammation.

Wanke, too, has reported considerable variations–between 3.5% and 85%–in the prevalence of duct abnormalities and dystopias [477].

2.3 Alcoholism

A history of alcohol abuse is very often found to be the precipitating cause (drinker's pancreatitis, pancreatitis after a heavy meal). At the autopsy of 51 patients who died in the course of acute alcohol intoxication, Weiner and Tenant [499] found an acute necrotizing pancreatitis to be the cause of death in 25 cases (49%).

Lehnert [283] is of the opinion that in about 90% of patients with alcoholic pancreatitis there have been preexisting pancreatic lesions, even if only of microscopic dimensions, due to the preceding chronic consumption of alcohol (for an average of 3–20 years). It must be assumed, therefore, that most cases represent an acute attack of a pancreatitis that had already been chronic (see Chapter 3).

2.4 Abdominal surgery: Postoperative pancreatitis

Acute pancreatitis can develop particularly after gastrointestinal operations (stomach, bile ducts, pancreas, spleen) and after operations on the transverse colon. However, it

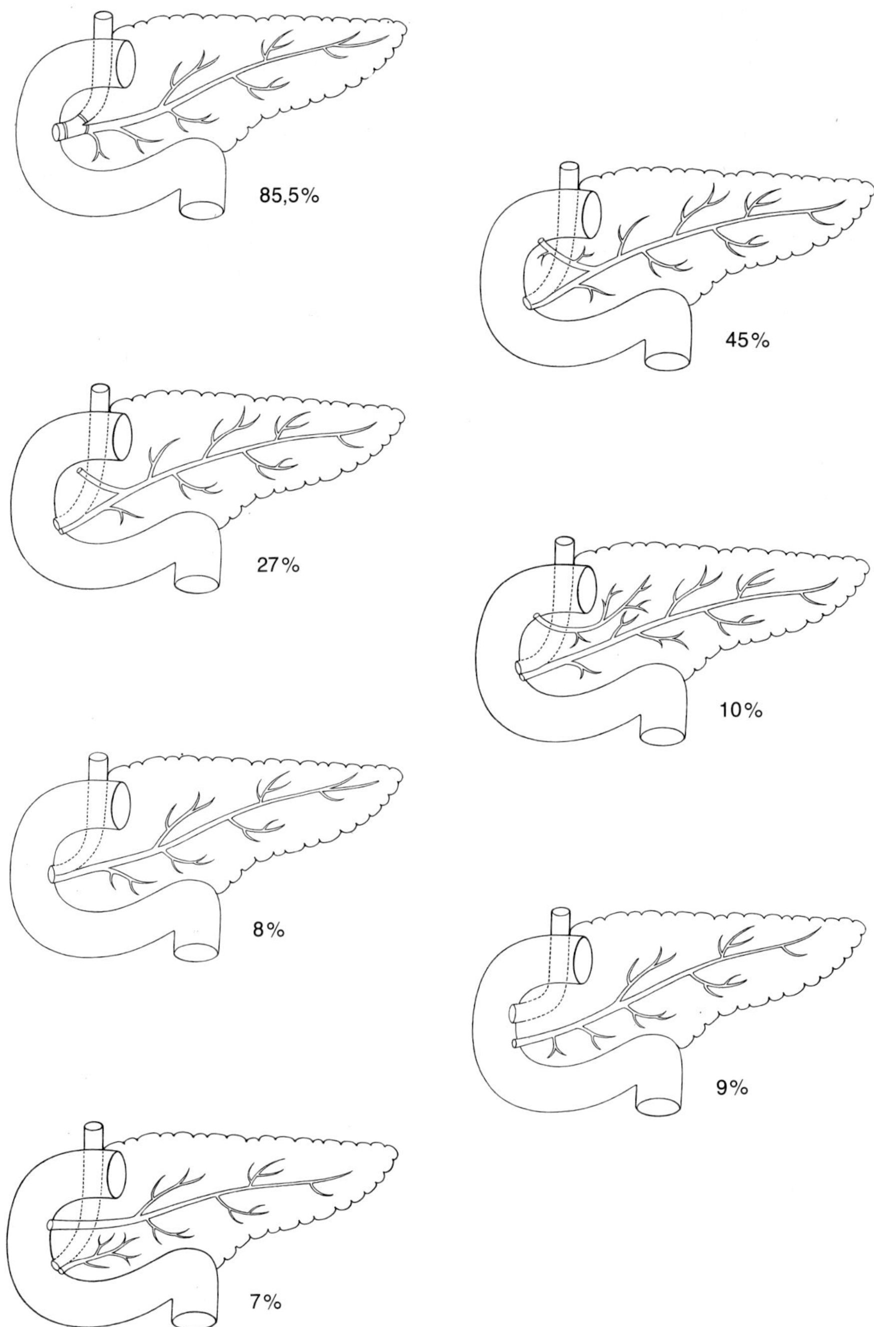

Fig. 1a. Prevalence of pancreatic duct anomalies.

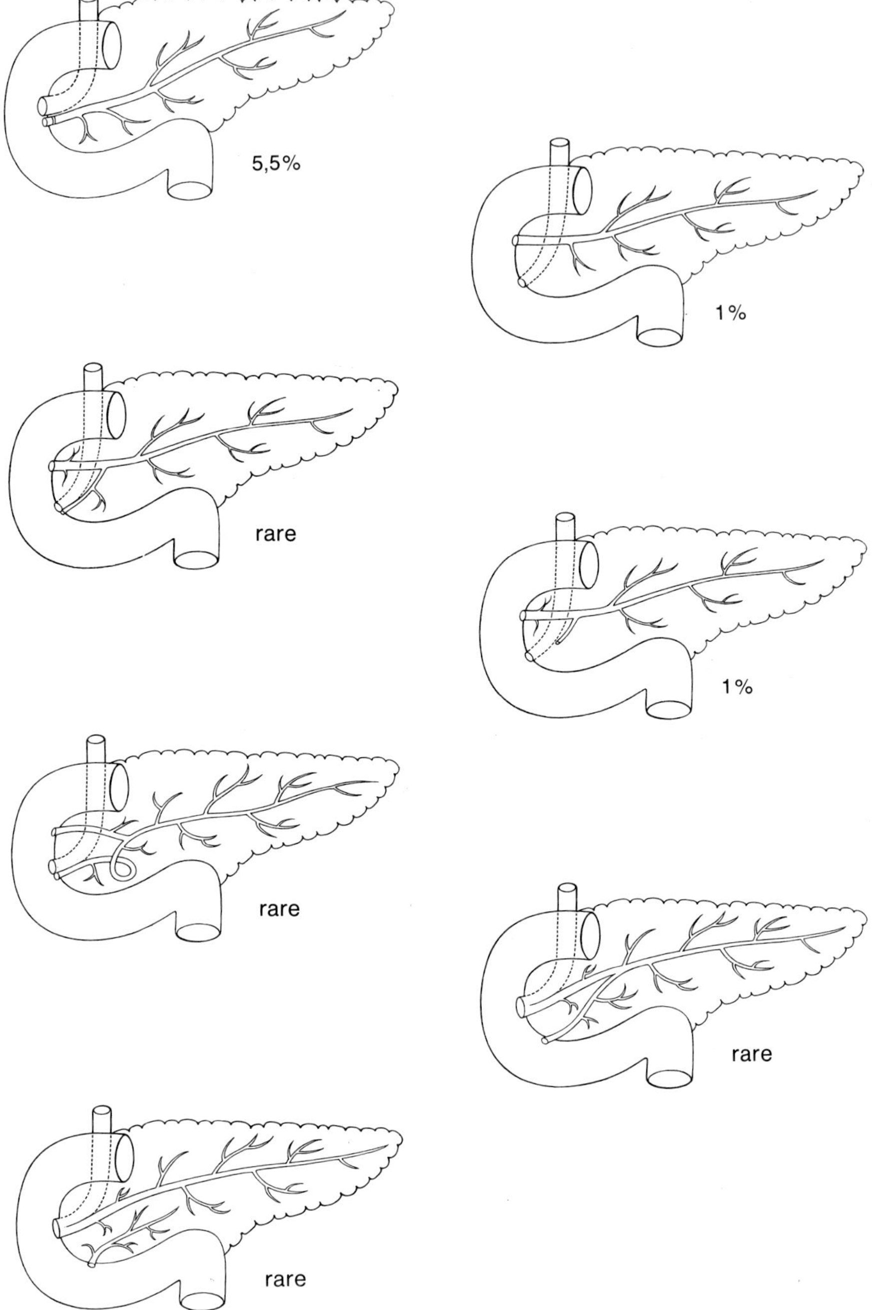

Fig. 1b. Prevalence of pancreatic duct anomalies.

Table 3. Possible causes of postoperative pancreatitis

I. Direct surgical traumas to the pancreas:
  a. Bile duct operations: Choledochotomy, bile duct repair, papillotomy, papillary trauma, duct ligation, wrong operative approach, resection of gastroduodenal ulcers penetrating the pancreas with devascularization due to ligation of vessels around head of pancreas
  b. Pancreatic surgery: Caudal pancreatectomy, corporocaudal pancreatectomy, isthmocorporocaudal pancreatectomy, subtotal pancreatectomy, duodenopancreatectomy (resection of pancreatic head), wirsingojejunal anastomoses, sclerosing of tail of pancreas, persistent pancreatolithiasis, drainage operation for pancreatic pseudocyst, pancreatic biopsies, injury to pancreas from resection of papilla, splenorenal anastomoses, splenectomy, gastrectomy

II. Indirect sequelae of surgery–effects on pancreas:
  Extensive mobilization with devascularization of head of pancreas following gastric resection (Billroth I – Billroth II), penetrating duodenal ulcer
  Duodenopancreatic reflux
  Afferent loop syndrome with duodenopancreatic reflux following gastric resection (Billroth II)
  Exacerbation of chronically relapsing pancreatitis

III. Indirect surgical traumas to the pancreas, traumatic effects on pancreas (sequelae of shock):
  Circulatory disorders, notably perioperative shock (due to blood loss), acidosis
  Protracted states of shock due to ileus, peritonitis
  Metabolic pancreatitis in uremia, diabetic coma (exacerbation of preexisting disease)
  Steroid therapy, endocrinopathies, e.g., surgery in hyperparathyroidism

---

can also be an indirect sequel of a wide variety of surgical procedures (Table 3).

Pancreatitis secondary to biliary tract surgery occurs chiefly after operations involving opening or exploration of the common bile duct and procedures in the region of the papilla. Transpapillary drainage with complete or incomplete compression of the orifice of the major pancreatic duct can also on occasion leed to acute pancreatitis, particularly in the absence of an accessory pancreatic duct (54% of cases according to Howard [222]).

The literature gives varying data regarding the percentages of acute pancreatitis following sphincterotomy and sphincteroplasty. Large-scale surveys generally yield a rate of 4%. We believe that the risk of pancreatitis after operations on the biliary tract and papilla is primarily due to traumatic, invasive operations on Oddi's sphincter. The region of the papilla is known to be a highly reflexogenic zone with a potential for neurovascular reactions.

Divergent reports have been given about the incidence of acute pancreatitis following gastric surgery. Rates of 0.5–1.5% have been cited. Billroth II gastric resection appears to provoke acute pancreatitis more frequently than Billroth I gastroduodenal anastomoses. In these cases, too, traumatic operation, overly deep incisions of the duodenum, or duodenal congestion with reflux into the pancreatic-biliary duct system are the chief pathogenetic factors.

Any operation on the pancreas itself can entail a postoperative acute pancreatitis. Particularly at risk are the resection stumps in the area of the pancreatic head and tail following partial duodenopancreatectomy. This is the so-called residual pancreatitis; its incidence has decreased since the introduction of the duct-sclerosing technique by

Ethiblock according to Gall and Gebhardt. Also to be borne in mind is the ever-present risk after pancreatic biopsy. The risk is decidedly greater after punch biopsy than after biopsy with a fine needle. Operations on organs adjoining the pancreas, and their consequences, have been repeatedly mentioned as indirect causes of postoperative pancreatitis. A chance coincidence cannot always be ruled out, however. It should also be noted that acute pancreatitis which may take a threatening course and end fatally has been observed in 5–6% of cases following open heart surgery, notably when this has been performed under hypothermia. Early diagnosis of such a postoperative pancreatitis is difficult, and therapy is rarely successful in preventing its onset [367].

2.4.1 Intraoperative endoscopy of biliary and pancreatic tracts

Choledochoscopy, choledochocholangiography, wirsungoscopy, retrograde wirsungography, sphincterotomy, and endoscopic papillotomy are operations that can pave the way for, or induce, acute pancreatitis. Mallet-Guy has shwon that this is attributable largely to the increased injection pressure of a column of more than 50–70 cm of water [299].

In actual practice, however, the extent of the risk may be presumed to be indirectly proportional to the operator's or endoscopist's experience during the operation. By way of example it may be noted that in the early phase of the introduction of endoscopic diagnostic and therapeutic procedures the incidence of ensuing pancreatitis was 5%–8%, whereas the risk today is reported to be less than 0.5% if the procedure is performed by experienced hands (see Chapter 6).

Numerous factors may contribute to the induction of postoperative pancreatitis. As a rule, a combination of several factors is involved:

Partial obstruction of pancreatic ducts by edema which is caused by more or less extensive manipulations at the papilla, by spasm of the sphincter of Oddi or the surrounding duodenal musculature, or by mechanical obstruction due to a drain or blood clot.

The vascular supply of the pancreas is compromised by operative ligatures, vasospasm, or systemically by an intraorperative or perioperative blood pressure drop and resultant metabolic acidosis.

There may also be a neurovascular reflex mechanism which could provoke vasoconstriction followed by vasodilation with focal hemorrhages into periacinar spaces. As in acidosis due to shock, proteolytic enzymes may then be released and activated by the metabolic damage and associated shift in pH. The possibility of an increase in the viscosity of pancreatic secretions under the action of certain drugs as well as of intracanalicular stasis of secretions due to partial mechanical or functional obstruction (e.g., of the afferent loop following Billroth II gastric resection) needs to be considered.

The problem of postoperative pancreatitis can be summed up in the statement: it is rare but dangerous [115].

The prognosis is poor and the mortality high, ranging up to 40% [65].

Likely pathogenetic factors, besides the necessarily close topographic relations, are the close functional relations between the pancreas and the organs adjoining it.

2.5   Pancreatitis and abdominal trauma

Any blunt injury to the pancreas associated with blunt abdominal trauma–which is more common than open, penetrating abdominal trauma–occurring alone or together with other traumata, can entail a so-called posttraumatic pancreatitis (Fig. 2).

2.5.1   General comments

The surgery of traumatically induced pancreatic lesions (posttraumatic pancreatitis) is a topic of timely significance for a number of reasons.

The growing number of diagnosed cases of posttraumatic pancreatitis is due to the increasing frequency of traffic accidents, on one hand, and to the increased rate of detection, on the other. This applies particularly to previously unrecognized cases of posttraumatic symptoms of initially uncomplicated pancreatitis following blunt abdominal trauma with or without associated injuries.

The possibility of injury or involvement of the pancreas needs to be considered whenever there is blunt abdominal injury, particular attention being paid to the possible development of posttraumatic pancreatitis in the subsequent clinical course (Fig. 2).

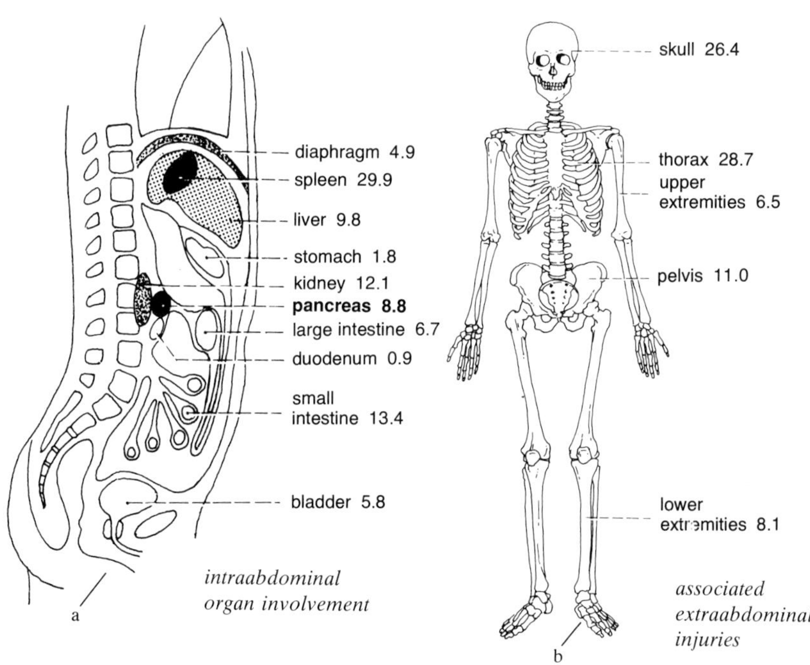

Fig. 2. Ratios (in percentages) of intraabdominal (a) and extraabdominal (b) *associated injuries* in 388 blunt abdominal traumas [336].

2.5.2 Types of injuries in pancreatic trauma

Instead of an isolated pancreatic lesion such as contusion of varying degrees and parenchymal or incomplete to complete ductal ruptures, multiple injuries are seen more and more frequently (see 2.5.5).

2.5.3 Distinctiveness of pancreatic trauma and posttraumatic pancreatitis

In terms of possible immediate and late complications of blunt abdominal trauma, the pancreas is distinguished from all the other organs in the abdominal cavity not only because of its retroperitoneal topographic situation but also because of its dual excretory and incretory glandular function, hence also its autodigestive capability.

2.5.4 Causes and mechanisms of injury

In blunt abdominal trauma, an exact reconstruction and analysis of the accident is of utmost importance for a rapid diagnosis concerning possible involvement of the pancreas. The transverse position of the organ in front of the vertebral column inevitably predisposes to certain types of injury and degrees of severity. Viewed mechanically, there may be direct violence to the spine as an abutment, or–which is far more common in grazing traffic injuries–trauma to a broad area with resultant compressive and shearing effects. The duct of Wirsung escapes injury in most cases owing to its elasticity and tortuous course.

2.5.5 Severity: Classification of pancreatic injuries

Degrees of severity are classified as follows–also with a view to appropriate surgical treatment–according to the varying extent of organ lesions and injuries:

Contusions of varying severity with or without parenchymal and ductal rupture:
Contusion (severity grade I): Neural and vascular irritation of organ without destruction of substance; simple contusion with ensuing edema, rarely hematoma; uncomplicated subsidence of edema.
Contusion (severity grade II): Morphologically determinable or sonographically detectable partial lesions of the organ with circumscribed detachments of capsule, capsule tears, subcapsular edema, and parenchymal hemorrhages with isolated areas of necrosis.

Parenchymal and ductal ruptures:
1. Subcapsular laceration without escape of pancreatic secretion, with capsule intact (possible rupture at two different times, involving healing of lesion and later pseudocyst formation).
2. Partial or incomplete tear of capsule and parenchyma extending as far as the intact pancreatic duct.
3. Total or complete parenchymal laceration with rupture of duct and division of organ in two (Fig. 3).

In all degrees of injury, the fact that an initially encapsulated hematoma is formed which may lead to incubation of blood and pancreatic secretions is of pathogenetic and pathophysiological significance. This may manifest itself locally by diffusion into the re-

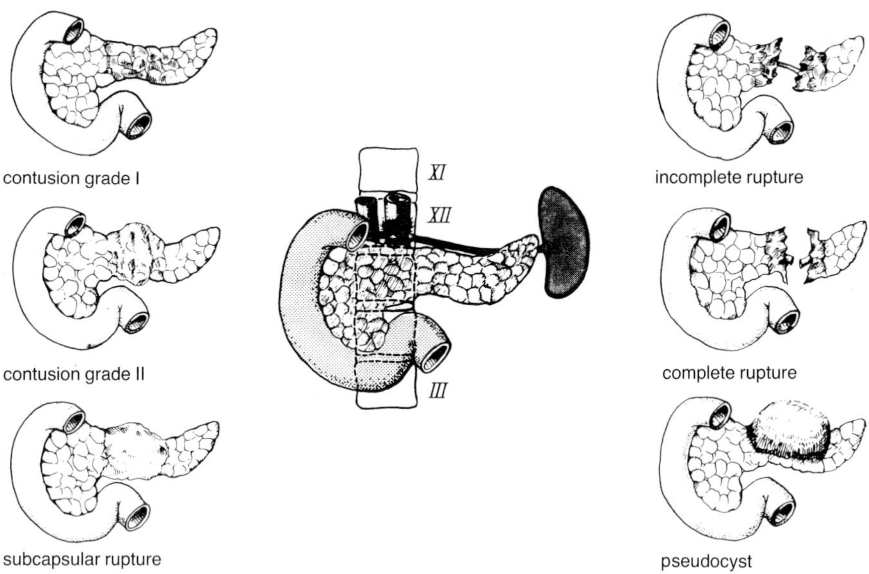

Fig. 3. Degrees of severity of pancreatic injuries [336].

troperitoneal connective tissue and the mesenteric septa and cause a general intoxication systemically.

In blunt abdominal trauma it is therefore always necessary to consider, apart from the abdominal and pancreatic injury per se, the possibility of traumatic or posttraumatic pancreatitis. Only thus can we prevent the success of a necessary or completed surgical intervention from being jeopardized by these early or late complications.

Late sequelae of pancreatic trauma: These comprise posttraumatic pancreatic fistulas and the development of posttraumatic pseudocysts. Not infrequently (in about 20% of all cases), pancreatic injuries that run an uncomplicated course manifest themselves several months afterward by the formation of a pseudocyst. The pathogenetic precondition for a pseudocyst is a previously incurred duct lesion or past pancreatitis.

Topographically, several cyst variants can develop: intrapancreatic, extrapancreatic-retroperitoneal, and extrapancreatic-intraperitoneal-parapancreatic pseudocysts.

2.6   Endocrinologic diseases and metabolic disorders

2.6.1   Hyperparathyroidism

Acute or chronic pancreatitis is found in about 7% of all patients with primary hyperparathyroidism [402]. In crises of hyperparathyroidism this percentage may even rise to 15–34% [161]. The frequency is so striking that a simple coincidence can be ruled out. Possible pathogenetic relationships are discussed in Chapter 3, Pathophysiology.

In chronic pancreatitis with a malassimilation syndrome, on the other hand, a secondary hyperparathyroidism may develop as a result of the reduced serum calcium level.

2.6.2 Pancreatitis of pregnancy and postpartum pancreatitis

Acute pancreatitis in pregnant women has been described, in both primigravidae and multigravidae or in multiparae, the reported incidence ranging from 0.002% to 0.026%. The problem of differential diagnosis then arises, i.e., the need to rule out so-called "obstetrical" shock (gestosis, eclampsia). A direct dependence of these forms of pancreatitis on the pregnancy can hardly be established even though some authors have reported finding a small increase of trypsin and lipase levels in the pancreatic juice toward the end of the pregnancy. Certain disturbances of corticosteroid metabolism are likely to be implicated.

Postpartum pancreatitis is exceedingly rare. We ourselves have seen 3 cases, 2 involving primiparae and 1 a multipara. The pancreatitis appeared 2−4 months after the delivery without the least sign of cholelithiasis. How these cases come about remains a mystery.

2.6.3 Pancreatitis in users of oral contraceptives

Whether oral contraceptives can provoke pancreatitis has not been clearly established. However, there is some evidence of it in the literature [34]. Clavadetscher and Weber found increased serum lipase activity in a group of more than 500 woman using oral contraceptives. Similar findings have been reported by Sommer, Krimmel, and Kasper. Conceivably, ovulation inhibitors can trigger pancreatitis through induction of hyperlipidemia [37, 73].

2.6.4 Hyperlipoproteinemias

Hyperlipoproteinemias can cause attacks of pancreatitis. Thus, cessation of pancreatic disorders has been observed after effective treatment of disorders of fat metabolism. It is a well-known fact that individuals with familial hyperlipoproteinemia often fall victim to acute pancreatitis (see Chapter 4) [61, 67].

2.7 Drugs as a cause of acute pancreatitis

A higher incidence of acute pancreatitis is seen after administration of thiazides, azathioprine and, especially, glucocorticoids.

2.7.1 Corticosteroids

The administration of corticosteroids, particularly in high doses, can provoke acute pancreatitis. Correlations of this type have been observed chiefly in children and in patients with nephrosis or acute nephritis who were being treated with prednisone or adrenocorticotropic hormone (ACTH) [55, 174]. Lindner has reported on 6 deaths due to acute pancreatitis among 115 patients with cirrhosis who had been treated with prednisone [289].

A metabolically induced pathogenetic mechanism may be assumed in the case of "cortisone pancreatitis" provoked by treatment with corticosteroids. Long-term administration of corticosteroids interferes with the functional metabolism and anabolism of the acinar cells and can result in dyschylia at an unforeseeable time. Of course, in many cases the underlying disease necessitating steroid therapy can be the principal etiological factor in the pancreatitis. It should also be borne in mind that any steroid therapy leads to a rise in neutral fat levels. Autoradiographic studies by Wanke et al. [492] support this conclusion inasmuch as adrenalectomized rats undergoing replacement therapy with hydrocortisone showed a significantly higher amino acid activity in the cytoplasm of the acinar cells than animals not so treated. Steroids, therefore, exert a regulatory effect on the enzyme pool of the acinar cells. This finding serves to elucidate the pathogenesis of so-called cortisone pancreatitis.

2.7.2   Other drugs

The concomitant onset of acute pancreatitis in connection with the administration of certain drugs (e.g., chlorothiazides, furosemide, cimetidine, azathioprine) has been described [300]. A critical review of these reports, however, shows that these are isolated instances and that the findings are not sufficient to prove a causal relationship.

2.8   Immunological and allergic factors causing pancreatitis

Theoretical considerations and animal study data [58, 253, 448] suggest that acute pancreatitis can be caused by an allergic mechanism. This also applies to acute pancreatitis observed in patients with rheumatism. It may be more of an inflammatory reaction accompanying the underlying rheumatoid disease.

According to Doerr, the allergic origin of acute pancreatitis may be assigned to one of three groups on the basis of experimental studies:
1. Induction of a serum, histamine, or peptone shock. Given the common vasculature of the liver and the pancreas, this results in serous pancreatitis.
2. Induction of an Arthus phenomenon: general sensitization; injection of allergen into the pancreatic duct or a pancreatic vein with ensuing hemorrhagic-necrotic inflammation.
3. Induction of a Shwartzman phenomenon.
From the point of view of general pathology, however, an overvaluation of such findings ought to be avoided [100, 101, 254].

2.9   Neurogenic pancreatitis

The following pathophysiological mechanisms may be considered as possible precipitating causes of a "neural pancreatitis": effect on pancreatic secretion; effect on the smooth musculature of the pancreatic duct-papillary system; and a vasoconstrictive effect causing disturbance of pancreatic blood flow, hypoxia and acidosis. However, the clinical significance of the pathogenetic and pathophysiological factors outlined above is as yet unproved [46, 159, 160].

2.10   Pancreatic reactions in circulatory and vascular diseases

The pancreas is attracting increasing clinical interest not only in the pathogenetic analysis of various gastroenterological diseases but also in cardiovascular diseases. Apart from posttraumatic sequelae and effects of shock on the pancreas, these are primary cardiovascular diseases and those which are detected only during, or because of, their chronic course (see Chapter 4). In a broader sense, this refers to reactions affecting the pancreas that are mediated by the circulatory system. We can understand this more readily if we consider the fact that an organ with so active a metabolism as the pancreas is particularly susceptible to all humoral and hemodynamic effects [335].

According to available published data, the following interrelations may enter into play, also in terms of differential diagnosis:

Cardiogenic effects or cardiovisceral correlations (coronary sclerosis/general ateriosclerosis with the special case of celiac stenosis [abdominal angina, malabsorption syndrome], malignant hypertension, portal hypertension).

General arteriosclerosis, as a systemic disease, does not spare the pancreas [41].

The question whether arteriosclerosis can play a role in pancreatic infarction has also been discussed in the literature. Nager and Steiner [338] described pancreatic infarction as the consequence of a sudden vascular occlusion in malignant hypertension. Hemodynamic and morphological changes in the venous leg of the pancreatic circulation may also predispose to the development of pancreatitis. Obstructive edema is observed in truncal portal vein thrombosis and sudden rise of portal pressure. Pathophysiologically, it is important to note that obstructive edema per se is not common since the transudation is more likely to ascites. On the other hand, such complications of a prior pancreatitis as ascites and pseudocyst formation, with or without pleural effusion, have to be differentiated (see Chapter 3 and the special case of segmental portal hypertension secondary to pancreatitis).

In addition, it should be noted that acute pancreatitis may develop whenever use is made of extracorporeal circulation in major heart surgery. Early diagnostic detection of this postoperative complication is difficult, and therapy is rarely successful in preventing it [367].

2.11   Hereditary pancreatitis

This form of pancreatitis is due to more serious metabolic disorders. Increased lysine and cystine and occasionally arginine levels in the urine have been demonstrated in more than half of the cases. The disease is transmitted in autosomal dominant fashion and is seen somewhat less frequently in women.

2.12   Viral pancreatitis

It has been thought for some time that pancreatic disease may also occur as a complication of mumps; according to some surveys it occurs in 2.4% of all cases of mumps. "Mumps pancreatitis" is characterized by epigastric pain and vomiting on the 3nd to 5th day after the swelling of the parotid. Several days after spontaneous healing of the parotitis the abdominal symptoms also subside. What is involved here is an interstitial inflammatory infiltration of the pancreas, preferentially caused by lymphocytes and plasma cells. Cases of hemorrhagic-necrotizing pancreatitis are exceptional [117, 284].

2.13   Parasitic pancreatitis

Cases of acute pancreatitis that were caused by Ascaris lumbricoides have been observed, with obstruction of the papilla, the common bile duct, or the duct of Wirsung. Such observations are not uncommon in countries with massive worm infestation.

2.14   Acute pancreatitis in children

Cases of acute pancreatitis in children are exceptional. The disease occasionally appears in connection with severe burns and, very rarely, with cholelithiasis or congenital malformation of the gallbladder or the pancreas (choledochal cyst, annular pancreas). Metabolic-toxic and traumatic factors as well as bacterial, viral, or parasitic infections are the predominant features in the pancreatitis of children (see 2.5.4 concerning post-traumatic pancreatitis in blunt abdominal trauma [475].

2.15   Idiopathic pancreatitis

This form of pancreatitis ranks fourth in incidence after cholecystocholedocholithiasis, alcoholism, and postoperative prancreatitis.

2.16   Ductal anomalies and pancreatitis

In a recently published paper, Cooperman et al. [77] reported on 35 cases of acute pancreatitis following retrograde cholangiopancreatography. In 16 of these 35 cases an anomaly in the ductal system or a malformation of the pancreas, papillary stenosis, pancreatic duct stenosis or lithiasis was discovered. Abnormalities can thus apparently promote the development of pancreatitis (Figs. 1a, 1b).

Chapter 3 – Pathophysiology

The individual factors described in Chapter 2, Etiology, can provoke acute pancreatitis by various pathogenetic mechnisms. On the other hand, a combination of several factors may be responsible for development of the disease in some cases.

3.1 Classification of acute pancreatitis according to pathogenesis and morphogenesis

Apart from some special and mixed forms, two main morphogenetic types can be distinguished: acute biliary reflux pancreatitis and acute lipolytic-proteolytic pancreatitis (see Chapter 4).

3.1.1 Biliary pancreatitis

The disease form produced by *reflux of bile* into the pancreatic duct system is associated with coagulation necrosis of ductal system epithelia and adjoining acinar cell complexes due to the detergent effect of the free bile acids. These primary lesions secondarily induce the release and activation of enzymes and autodigestion (Fig. 4, Plate I). The primary cause is choledocholithiasis. The divergent numerical data given on the frequency with which cholelithiasis causes acute pancreatitis (approximately 40–50%), on one hand, and on the detection of an impacted papillary stone (1–5%), biliary reflux pancreatitis (6%), or choledocholithiasis (10%), on the other hand, are worth noting [160] (see Chapter 2). An interim (and frequently demonstrable) discharge of the calculus may explain the variability of these data [3, 323]. The fact that there is usually no recurrence of pancreatitis after cholecystectomy argues against the assumption that a chance concurrence of cholelithiasis and acute pancreatitis offers the best explanation (see Chapter 2).

Hess [186] and Neumayr and Peschl [341], moreover, assume a causal relation between cholecystitis and pancreatitis in the sense of a *lymphogenous* transmission of a "cholecystopancreatitis" or satellite pancreatitis from the inflamed gallbladder to the head of the pancreas (Fig. 4, Plate I).

3.1.2 Acute lipolytic-proteolytic pancreatitis

This also leads to release and activation of enzymes via the stages of pancreatic juice edema, disturbed circulation, and acidosis, and to autodigestion (Fig. 4, Plate I). The chief etiological factors to be mentioned are metabolic and toxic causes. This group presumably also encompasses so-called idiopathic pancreatitis.

3.1.3   Chyme reflux pancreatitis

This is a mixed form of pancreatitis combining the biliary reflux and lipolytic-proteolytic types.

Infectious pancreatitides are classified as special morphogenetic disease forms.

3.2   "Precursory phase"

The morphological and functional pancreatic changes subsumed under the term "precursory phase," which are induced particularly by alimentary, toxic, hormonal, and metabolic factors, promote the development of acute pancreatitis and are demonstrable in 85 % of patients with acute lipolytic-proteolytic pancreatitis (see Chapter 4 and Fig. 4, Plate I).

To be mentioned, above all, are intra- and peripancreatic proliferation of adipose tissue, adipositas interna, vascular sclerosis, periductular and interlobular fibrosis with lymphatic vessel obliteration and resultant lymph blockade and stasis of pancreatic juice ("chronic pancreatitis en miniature"). To be noted particularly are obesity, disorders of fat metabolism and age-related vascular changes (see Chapters 2 and 4).

The functional and morphological changes observed with *chronic alcohol consumption,* which are produced by independent pathophysiological mechanisms, should also be cited in a discussion of the precursory phase of pancreatitis even though alcoholic pancreatitis should be classified among chronic-progressive forms in the great majority of cases [283]. In the initial stage of the disease in particular, these changes strongly promote the provocation of an acute attack of pancreatitis [129].

Comparative functional and morphological studies by Sarles et al. [402] have shown that formation of a protein-rich secretion with subsequent precipitation of proteins in the pancreatic duct system is the point of departure for the chronic alterations of the pancreas.

In contrast to a one-time administration of alcohol, which leads to a decrease in exocrine pancreatic secretion, an increase of protein secretion by the pancreas which sets in after about 6 weeks and remains detectable for several months occurs upon chronic administration of alcohol and, concomitantly, of a high-fat and high-protein diet in animal studies. Long-term studies in dogs have shown that after prolonged administration of alcohol (2–3 years) the secretion of protein diminishes and water and bicarbonate secretion increases. Both effects are attributed to an increased cholinergic tone of the pancreas. Individuals with a chronic daily consumption of more than 150 ml of pure alcohol who did not suffer from clinically overt pancreatic disease were also found to have a significantly higher basal concentration than normal persons [283, 402]. Lactoferrin, which can bind acid proteins besides iron, is increased in the pancreatic secretions of patients with chronic pancreatitis. This could promote the precipitation of proteins in the pancreatic secretion [326].

Ca^{++} deposits on the protein precipitates so formed, and stone formation and calcification result. Owing to the chronic mechanical irritation they produce, these protein precipitates and concrements cause atrophy of the ductal epithelium, later proliferation of pericanalicular connective tissue, and finally ductal stenoses and occlusions and a consequent pressure rise in the pancreatic duct system; in the end the secretion is accomplished only "against resistance."

According to rat studies by Jalovaara [233], *chronic* administration of alcohol shifts the ratio of the concentrations of trypsin inhibitor and protein (enzymes) in the pancreatic secretion toward a lower inhibitor content, as a result of which premature activation of the zymogens may be abetted. The presence of high enzyme levels has also been ascribed to premature activation of chymotrypsinogen by traces of free trypsin, not only in relation to the provocation of acute attacks of pancreatitis but also with respect to the formation of protein precipitates [401]. Furthermore, it has been suggested that a direct toxic effect of alcohol and a hypersecretory-obstructive mechanism may be the cause of the onset of acute pancreatitis or of an acute attack of chronic pancreatitis [329]. Besides the aforementioned morphological alterations of the pancreas, papillary edema, papillary spasm, and obstructive duodenitis have been considered as possible obstacles to outflow, and gastrin and gastric acid–besides the increased cholinergic tone–as causes of the hypersecretion. In addition, rises in intraduodenal pressure due to frequent vomiting could perhaps induce acute pancreatitis by reflux of duodenal contents into the pancreatic duct system (bile, activated enzymes, chyme) [283].

Acute or chronic pancreatitis has been described in 7% of patients with *primary hyperparathyroidism* and characterized as acute pancreatitis in about one-half of these cases [399]. Under basal conditions as well as after secretin stimulation, acute hypercalcemia (infusion of Ca^{++}) leads to an increase of enzyme concentration and enzyme secretion which can be inhibited by means of atropine. The hydrokinetic function of the pancreas is unaffected by hypercalcemia. At the same time, the Ca^{++} concentration in the pancreatic secretion is markedly increased. In about one-half of cases of chronic hypercalcemia due to primary hyperparathyroidism, pancreatic enzyme secretion is already reduced [161].

Just as in pancreatitis induced by chronic alcohol consumption, the pathoanatomical changes in this disease form caused by chronic hypercalcemia originate from protein precipitates in the pancreatic duct system. Thus, increased protein concentrations in the pancreatic secretion with ensuing protein precipitation in the ductal system have been produced in animal experiments by parenteral administration of Ca^{++} [399]. The pathogenesis of chronic pancreatitis in the presence of hypercalcemia thus conforms to that in chronic alcohol abuse. This promotes the development of acute pancreatitis ("precursory phase") in a similar fashion.

Intrapancreatic activation of trypsinogen by high Ca^{++} concentrations and a toxic effect of the hypercalcemia or–which is not very likely–of the excess of parathyroid hormone have been considered as possible causes of acute pancreatitis or an acute attack of chronic pancreatitis [161]. The high concomitant incidence of acute pancreatitis (25–34%) during a crisis of hyperparathyroidism should also be mentioned in this connection [138]. The fact that acute pancreatitis can also be induced by hypercalcemia due to other causes (e.g., vitamin D intoxication) underscores the pathophysiological significance of elevated Ca^{++} levels [161].

3.3   Autodigestion and inflammation

The release and activation of enzymes and autodigestion are focal points of acute hemorrhagic-necrotizing pancreatitis. The pancreas has numerous protective factors for their prevention. So long as these predominate, the pathoanatomical changes of the pancreas produce no clinical symptoms (with normal as well as pathological laboratory findings), or lead to edematous pancreatitis only. If the aggressive factors predominate, on the other hand, the severe disease form, acute hemorrhagic-necrotizing pancreatitis, develops; this is detectable by laboratory investigations, sonography, and computed tomography. Its extent is in proportion to the imbalance of aggressive and protective factors (see Chapter 4).

Protective factors (Chapter 4) to be singled out are the synthesis of proteolytic enzymes and phospholipases as inactive precursors (zymogens), their isolation from the cytosol by membranes during transport and storage in the acinar cells (zymogen granules), and the supply of protease inhibitors in the acinar cells, in the pancreatic secretions and the serum (see below). Another factor is the unimpeded efflux of secretions from the ductal system and the possibility of parapedesis with undisturbed lymph drainage (see Chapter 4).

In the *activation of zymogens* trypsin plays a central role since it not only autocatalytically activates trypsinogen to trypsin but activates all the other pancreatic zymogens (chymotrypsinogen, proelastase, prekallikrein, procarboxypeptidases, prephospholipases) as well. Traces of free trypsin appear to suffice for the activation process. Free trypsin could form unter certain conditions (acidosis, hypercalcemia, shift away from inhibitor in ratio of trypsinogen and inhibitor concentrations in the pancreas) not only by autocatalysis in the zymogen granules but also by activation by lysosomal enzymes [129]. A possible activation of trypsinogen by thrombin and plasmin has also been suggested in this connection [16]. Furthermore, trypsin activated by enteropeptidase in the duodenum could enter the pancreas in the event of a reflux of duodenal contents.

A *specific trypsin inhibitor* is synthesized in the pancreas and secreted together with the enzymes or zymogens for the purpose of preventing a premature activation of trypsin. This forms reversible equimolar complexes with trypsin (dissociation at pH <5) [136].

The tissue-based trypsin inhibitor which Kunitz and Northrop demonstrated in cattle in 1936 does not occur in man. Besides trypsin, it binds chymotrypsin, plasmin, and especially kallikrein, and for this reason it had been discovered as a "kallikrein inactivator" 6 years before by Frey, Kraut, and Werle [98, 135]. This trypsin-kallikrein inhibitor, detected in various other organs of cattle as well, is used therapeutically as aprotinin (Trasylol®) (see Chapter 10).

In addition to the specific trypsin inhibitor, *nonspecific protease inhibitors* in the plasma and serum play an important role in the inactivation of trypsin, kallikrein, and other proteases. According to studies by Balldin et al. [29, 30] performed in dogs in vivo and in vitro, active trypsin is bound in the plasma mainly to α_2-macroglobulin. Binding to α_1-antitrypsin seems to be of secondary importance. The latter is credited only with a carrier function.

The binding of trypsin by α_2-macroglobulin does not, however, lead to complete inhibition of the proteolytic activity of this enzyme. While the proteolytic activity of the protease-α_2-macroglobulin complex is abolished for proteins of higher molecular weight, it seems to persist for lower molecular weight ester and amide compounds and peptides (e.g., peptide hormones such as parathyroid hormone, vasopressin, angiotensin II, and proinsulin) [60]. This residual proteolytic activity, too, can be inhibited by aprotinin [33]. However, aprotinin has less affinity for this complex than for free trypsin. On the other hand, trypsin has a greater affinity for α_2-macroglobulin than for aprotinin, and for this reason the latter is able to bind and inactivate free trypsin only after the available free α_2-macroglobulin has been used up.

Trypsin contributes to the induction of pancreatogenous shock not only indirectly, by activation of prekallikrein and subsequent kinin release, but can also directly split off bradykinin from kininogen. Thus, dog studies in vivo and in vitro by Balldin et al. [29] have shown that infusions of trypsin after saturation of available α_2-macroglobulin lead to release of bradykinin and, consequently, to shock. Concomitant administration of aprotinin inhibits this effect [32].

Besides elevated lipase, amylase and phospholipase A levels, an increase of radioimmunologically measured trypsin concentrations is observed in the serum of patients with acute pancreatitis (see Chapter 6). According to studies by Brodrick et al. [59], both trypsinogen and trypsin bound to α_2-macroglobulin and α_1-antitrypsin account for this increase. Possible binding to other, nonspecific, protease inhibitors or to the specific trypsin inhibitor was not considered in these studies.

Free proteases such as trypsin, chymotrypsin, and elastase were detected in the pancreatic exudate of dogs with experimental biliary pancreatitis in the early stage of the disease in addition to the proteases bound to α_2-macroglobulin and α_1-antitrypsin [350, 490]. High ascitic fluid levels of phospholipase, lipase and amylase have also been noted in patients with acute hemorrhagic-necrotizing pancreatitis [343]. Furthermore, proteases (trypsin, elastase) bound to α_2-macroglobulin or α_1-antitrypsin have also been detected in the ascitic fluid of such patients [31].

3.4 Pathophysiological effects of pancreatic enzymes

3.4.1 Local pancreatic alterations

These changes in adjoining organs, like the systemic changes, in acute pancreatitis are not induced by a single enzyme alone. They result from the sum total of direct and indirect enzymatic effects. Nonetheless, animal study data on the injurious effects of individual enzymes point to pathophysiological interrelations (Table 4, Fig. 4, Plate I). The specific cellular substrates of the liberated pancreatic enzymes and the pathoanatomical changes they produce in the pancreas are described in Chapter 4 (specifically, Table 15).

Table 4. Pathophysiological effects of enzymes and toxic substances released in acute pancreatitis (from Nevalainen [343])

Substance	Effect (direct or indirect)
Trypsin	Shock, proteolysis, coagulopathies, kinin release
Chymotrypsin	Proteolysis
Elastase	Proteolysis, elastolysis, hemorrhages
Lipase	Adipose tissue necrosis, hypocalcemia
Phospholipase A	Hydrolysis of phospholipids, lysolecithin formation, shock lung
Kallikrein	Kinin release
Kinins and histamine	Edema, pain, shock due to vasodilation, increase of permeability ("permeation")
Myocardial depressant factor	Reduction of cardiac output, additional adverse effect on circulatory status

3.4.2   Adipose tissue necrosis

In the vicinity of the pancreas, adipose tissue necrosis is caused in the presence of bile salts by pancreatic lipase, phospholipase A, and the triglyceride lipase of adipose tissue. Incorporation of Ca^{++} leads to the familiar "calcium splashes."

Enzyme release and enzyme activation not only cause autodigestion and local complications but can also have direct or indirect systemic effects by liberating kinins, histamine, and other toxic substances [16, 227, 456].

3.4.3   Shock and pain

Besides hypovolemia due to hemorrhagic ascites and exudation, intra- and peripancreatic edema, retroperitoneal fluid and blood loss, and ileus, vasoactive substances must be directly involved in the shock process. Within the first few minutes, as a matter of fact, after induction of an experimental acute hemorrhagic-necrotizing pancreatitis a blood pressure drop is observed, which is transmissible to other animals by cross-perfusion [12, 128]. Kinins cause vasodilation and increase of vascular permeability with stasis, thromboses and hemorrhages, and provoke pain. Inasmuch as kinins are biologically inactivated very quickly, they act mostly at their site of formation. Besides kinins, histamine can be released by destruction of cell membranes (phospholipases), and this likewise leads to increased vascular permeability and a blood pressure drop. The pain is attributable in part to the kinin action and in part to the edema-induced capsule tension, which explains the great intensity of the pain even in edematous pancreatitis. Yet the findings made by palpation are at first not so severe owing to the retroperitoneal, anatomically encapsulated pancreatic compartment (see Chapters 5, 7, 8).

3.4.4   Remote systemic effects

The systemic effects of the released active enzymes can directly or indirectly (kinins, histamine, shock) entail remote complications in the lungs, kidneys, liver, heart, and brain, in blood coagulation, and in the electrolyte, carbohydrate and lipid metabolism [456, 472, 484]. The most important data are presented in Table 5 (see also Chapter 4).

3.4.5   Hypocalcemia

The hypocalcemia observed in severe cases is probably due to several causes. Besides calcium deposits in the necrotized adipose tissue (see above), they are: reduced parathyroid hormone levels due to the cleavage by pancreatic proteases [60]; release of calcitonin by glucagon [161]; decrease of protein-bound Ca^{++}; and shifting of extracellular and intracellular Ca^{++} concentrations [227].

3.4.6   Hypophosphatemia

Hypophosphatemia associated with increased phosphate excretion has been reported in acute pancreatitis by Jacobson et al. [232] and ascribed to reduced tubular reabsorp-

Table 5. Systemic effects and consequences of release of enzymes, kinins, and toxic substances in acute pancreatitis

Substrate	Effect
Vessels/perivascular space/heart	Shock, thromboembolism, erosive hemorrhages, ascites, pleural or pericardial effusion, ischemia
Lung	Shock lung
Stomach/intestine	Erosions/ulcers, subileus/ileus
Liver/biliary tract/spleen	Shock necrosis, dystrophy, cholestasis, icterus, compression of common bile duct by pancreatic edema or pseudocysts in region of head, segmental portal hypertension (due to pancreatic edema, pseudocysts)
Kidneys	Shock kidneys Necrotizing nephrosis
Adipose tissue	Ubiquitous necroses
Brain	Pancreatic encephalopathy
Metabolism	Disturbances of electrolyte metabolism (e.g., hypocalcemia, hypophosphatemia, hypokalemia), Hyperlipoproteinemia, hyperglycemia/diabetes, hypalbuminemia
Coagulation	Hyper- and hypocoagulopathies

tion. Inasmuch as cerebral states of disorientation have been described in connection with reduced serum phosphate levels, the discovery of hypophosphatemia, with subsequent phosphate replacement therapy, takes on particular significance in acute pancreatitis.

3.4.7 Hyperglycemia

Hyperglycemia accompanying acute pancreatitis is caused not only by destruction of islet cells but also by changes in the control variables (absolute or relative increase of glucagon levels, stress-induced increases of cortisol and catecholamines), or else by preexisting diabetes [251], (Fig. 5).

3.4.8 Hyperlipoproteinemia

Familial hyperlipoproteinemia can be the cause of acute pancreatitis. On the other hand, acute pancreatitis itself can bring about an increase of the serum lipid concentrations through increased lipolysis. Finally, chronic alcohol abuse can provoke pancreatitis as well as secondary hyperlipoproteinemia. Observation of the course will permit a differentiation [291].

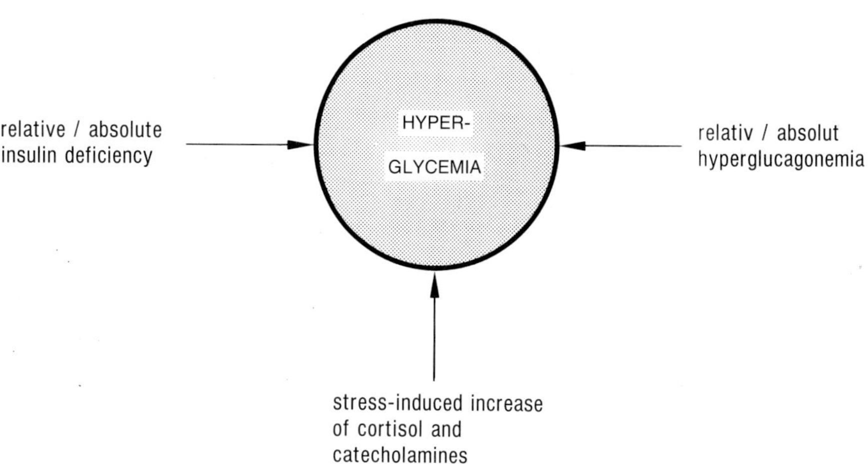

Fig. 5. Causes of hyperglycemia in acute pancreatitis (Klose et al. [251]).

3.4.9   Pleural and pericardial effusions, ascites

These, as well as inflammatory intraperitoneal and retroperitoneal exudations, are frequent complications and side effects of acute pancreatitis. Besides a local enzyme effect associated with hemorrhage and necrosis, blockade of the cisterna chyli is believed responsible for the development of ascites [333]. Pleural and pericardial effusions are, as a rule, of lymphogenous origin but may also be provoked hematogenously. The possibility of a continuous spread of the inflammation (across the diaphragm owing to increased permeability or fistulas), particularly in left-sided pleural effusion, has also been considered. Here again, kinins and histamine are of pathophysiological importance; right-sided pleural effusions are primarily due to cardiovascular causes (Fig. 6).

3.5   Approaches to the therapy of acute pancreatitis

Three main pathophysiological approaches to a specific therapy of acute pancreatitis (apart from general measures and intensive care, notably fluid and electrolyte replacement and shock management) can be derived from the available pathophysiological data and demonstrable interrelations (see Chapters 10 and 11):

1. Reduction of secretory pressure (e.g., depressing activity of the gland by abstinence from food, by somatostatin) and assurance of free outflow of secretion (e.g., endoscopic papillotomy in choledocholithiasis with congestion of bile ducts and pancreatic duct).

2. Earliest possible use of enzyme inhibitors (e.g., aprotinin, Trasylol®).

3. Removal of toxic substances from the body (therapeutic peritoneal lavage, surgical intervention).

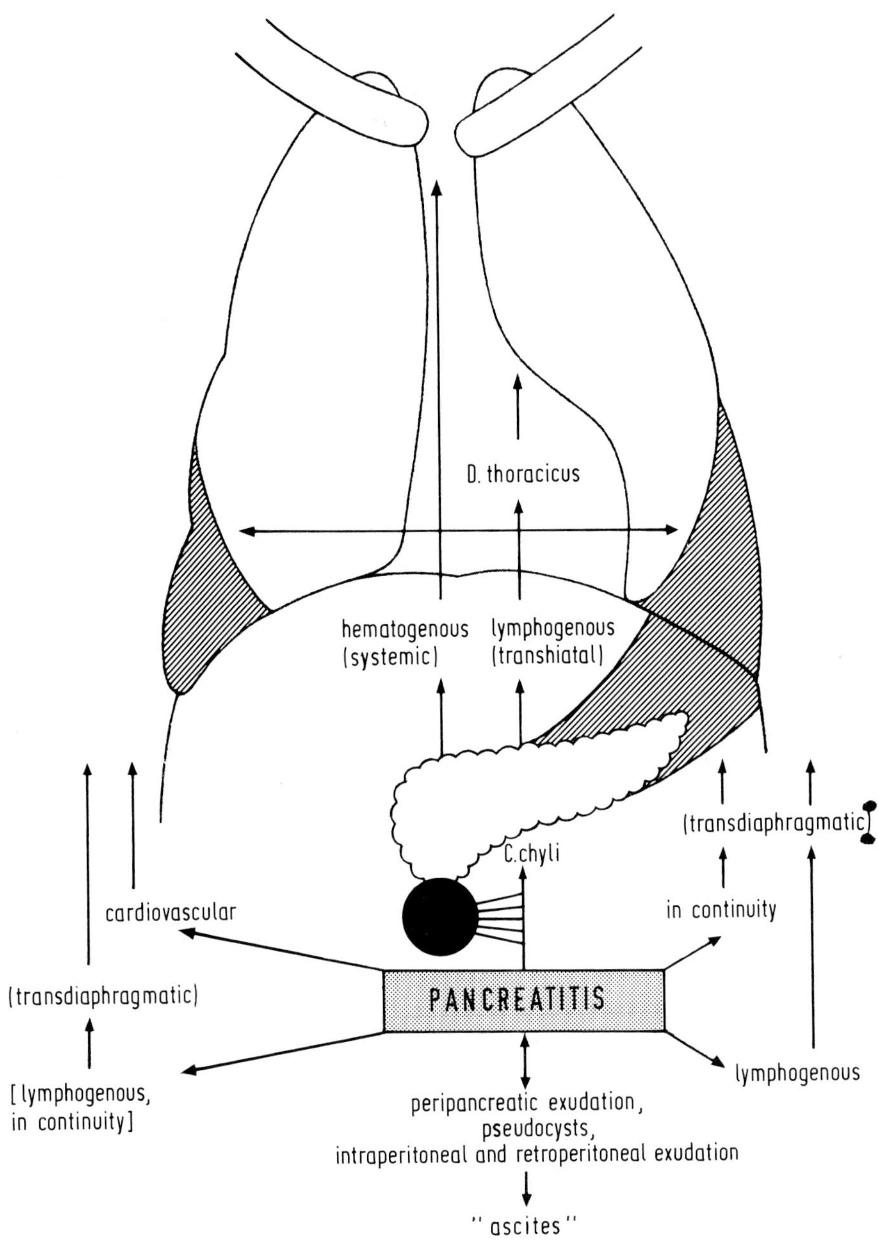

Fig. 6. Possible causes of pleural and pericardial effusions in acute pancreatitis (Nagel 1973).

Chapter 4 – Pathogenesis and Morphogenesis

4.1 Introduction

Initial descriptions of acute pancreatitis date back to Bonetus, 1664, and to Morgagni, 1761. The components characterizing the morphological picture, such as necrosis of adipose tissue and parenchyma with or without hemorrhages, sequestration, and calcification were recognized as important even by Portal in 1811, Claessen in 1842, and Klebs in 1876.

Zenker reported in 1874 on pancreatic hemorrhages as the cause of sudden death. Balser wrote, in 1882, about adipose tissue necrosis, an occasionally fatal disease of man, and Chiari, in 1895, about autodigestion of the human pancreas. In 1966 Wanke drew a morphological distinction between biliary, lipolytic, and proteolytic forms of acute pancreatitis.

The morphogenetic significance of the hemorrhagic component ("hemorrhagic pancreatitis") and its prognostic significance in individual cases were debated by Fitz in 1889, Körte in 1894, and Hahn in 1901 and are still being debated today.

We know from Heidenhain since 1875 that the proteolytic enzymes of the pancreas are present in the acinar cells as inactive zymogens. Only the action of "acid" on the acinar cell makes possible "enzymatic action in the wrong place"–autodigestion. According to our present knowledge, based on experimental studies and analysis of clinical and autopsy observations about the central role of acidosis [471, 472, 480] in zymogen activation, Heidenhain's concept remains valid even today. Hildebrand (1895) must be regarded the actual originator of the "enzyme theory" of the genesis of pancreatitis; he surmised that the joint action of steapsin (lipase) and trypsin was the cause of the organ's necrosis. Hess (1903) questioned at the beginning of the century the "toxic effect" of trypsin, viewing instead the "soaps" liberated by the hydrolysis of lipase (cf. local acidosis following triglyceride cleavage by lipase [468, 469, 480]) as the determining pathogenetic principle. In 1909 Hess succeeded in experimentally inducing hemorrhagic pancreatitis in the dog by intraductular instillation of lecithin (contaminated with lysolecithin). Shortly before, in 1907, Friedmann had isolated a substance from the pancreas that was able to form hemolysins susceptible to activation by lecithin. These findings may be considered as forerunners of the "phospholipase A-lysolecithin" concept of the genesis of parenchymal necrosis [343].

Observations by Opie in 1901 about the more than accidental frequency of the coincidence of cholelithiasis and pancreatitis (Table 6), and by Halsted in 1901 about the effect of bile reflux into the pancreatic duct in the presence of a "common channel" (common terminal course of choledochous duct and duct of Wirsung, 5–10 mm long, before opening into papilla of Vater) after papillary stone impaction as the cause of acute pancreatitis (pancreatic apoplexy!), subsequently overshadowed past experience regarding different aspects of the "pancreatitis disease."

There have been repeated attempts until quite recently to differentiate pancreatitis and pancreatic necrosis [362]. If the concept of inflammation is interpreted morphogenetically, such a differentiation is inappropriate, according to Doerr [100] from the pathoanatomical viewpoint. However, the experience underlying the two concepts is that there is one group of pancreatitides that can be shown to have resulted from bacterial, parasitic, or viral infections (see 4.6) and exhibit a decidedly duct-related, purulent component, and another group presenting the morphologically nearly specific substrate of autodigestive or biliary organ destruction with a "secondary inflammatory character."

There is, on the other hand, a widely held desire to arrive at a monocausal interpretation of a disease pattern; thus, in 1965 Pincus, among others (quoted by Wanke [469]), ascribed all the manifestations of acute pancreatitis to a "basic process" while conceding the presence of various accessory factors.

The idea of a common pathogenetic basis of all forms of acute pancreatitis appears to be supported by the experience that they start almost invariably with edema (vascular or due to dyschylia). It should be stated at once that the danger of vascular edema is not comparable to that of dyschylous edema! Thus, the ensuing clinical course may end in full remission (majority of so-called associated pancreatitides), or it may be characterized by recurrent microlesions of the type of lipolytic-proteolytic "minimal lesions," or it may culminate in the great catastrophy of pancreatic apoplexy in biliary pancreatitis. According to this conception, there is seemingly only a quantitative difference, not a qualitative one, between the individual forms of pancreatitis. Yet if we try to match etiology, pathogenesis, and morphogenesis, we find that the proposed concept cannot be sustained.

The morphological differentiation of biliary and autodigestive lipolytic-proteolytic pancreatitis reveals that in the majority (approximately 85%) of acute pancreatitis cases the ground has been prepared for it and it runs a phasizing course [472], whereas the hemorrhagic-necrotizing form, accounting for about 15%, is due in 6% of the cases to bile reflux with a common channel, 3% thereof having an impacted papillary stone [186] not counting transient stone impaction (see Chapter 3, [3, 323]) and in another 9% to massive reflux of chyme [309], and has a characteristic history related to food intake (see Chapter 5). The confusion about the pathogenesis of acute pancreatitis is mainly attributable to the failure to make a clear distinction between etiological factors and the mechanism by which these cause pancreatitis.

The simple *distinction* between a *biliary* and a *nonbiliary cause* and characterization of the stages of the disease course as edematous or hemorrhagic-necrotizing with partial or total organ necrosis have in most cases proved satisfactory for clinical-therapeutic purposes. However, despite numerous comparative studies presented in the world literature, this rough classification as yet allows no definitive conclusion to be drawn favoring an active conservative as contrasted with a surgical approach since the patients, diagnostic procedures, choice of operative technique, and the evaluation of disease severity were not comparable in the various studies.

The pathogenesis and morphological substrates of acute pancreatitis allow us to distinguish a primarily nonenzymatic biliary pancreatitis (BP) from an autodigestive lipolytic-proteolytic variant (LPP), disregarding any special forms for the present:

Pathogenesis

1. Canalicular	Biliopancreatic reflux
	Chymopancreatic reflux
2. Vascular	Arteriosclerotic
	Arteritic
	Shock

3. Traumatic   Exogenous

                                     Iatrogenic-postoperative

4. Metabolic   Polyadenomatosis

   a. Dyschylia   Hypercorticism, hyperparathyroidism, pregnancy

   b. Acidosis   Uremia, alcoholism

   c. Hyperlipoproteinemia   Undernourishment, malnutrition, hyperlipemia

5. Idiopathic   ?

6. Special forms   Viral, bacterial, parasitic infections

Morphogenesis

BP: The fulminant hemorrhagic-necrotizing, primarily nonenzymatic biliary form (BP) runs a "single-phase" course. Initial reflux-related coagulation necrosis of ductal tree epithelia and disseminated acinar complexes are the result of the detergent effect of unconjugated bile acids; the edema is initially of vascular origin.

LPP: The autodigestive lipolytic-proteolytic type (LPP) develops in phases (prephase, trigger phase, postphase) via the morphological stages of dyschylia, pancreatic juice edema, disturbed circulation, necrobiosis, and autodigestion. Accordingly, the macroscopic organ findings are characterized by edema, necrosis of adipose tissue and parenchyma, and hemorrhages.

MP: Mixed forms of acute pancreatitis (MP) develop after reflux of chyme; in these cases the morphological finding of organ necrosis is stamped from the beginning by a biliary and enzymatic-autodigestive component; by the same token, the edema is of a mixed vascular-dyschylous type from the outset.

IP: Infectious pancreatitides (IP) are a special form intermediate between the chemical (BP) and autodigestive (LPP) forms: the mesenchymal reaction involving the vascular-connective tissue apparatus predominates, presenting the typical equivalents of acute inflammation, viz., serous, seropurulent, purulent, purulent/abscess-forming, and hemorrhagic.

Within the context of the "pancreatitic disease" it is necessary to distinguish between the local alterations in the pancreas itself and the general consequences of the enzyme derangement for vessels and perivascular space, adipose-connective tissue, and the great parenchymatous organs (Fig. 4, Plate I [476, 480, 482, 484, 490]).

4.2   Comparative pathology

All forms of acute and chronic pancreatitis occurring in humans are also seen in the animal kingdom [239]. Whether adipose tissue and parenchymal necrosis or hemorrhages predominate depends on the enzyme pattern of the affected species and on the topical relationships between the pancreatic duct and the common bile duct; besides, nutritional habits (omnivorous, carnivorous, or herbivorous) have an important effect on the quantitative ratio among the pancreatic enzymes [44, 98] as well as on endocrine factors [486, 492]. The pancreatic juice of cattle, as herbivores, contains only traces of lipase, for example, whereas in the omnivorous pig lipase accounts for 6.5% of pancreatic enzymes [342]; accordingly, one never sees the disease picture, or makes the finding of chronic or acute pancreatitis in cattle despite the fact that sialolithiasis is a common occurrence in this species [239] (Fig. 7, Plate II); only in fattened calves with considerable adipose tissue infiltration of the pancreas is fat necrosis demonstrable. These findings are comparable to the rarity of acute pancreatitis in children [473, 475].

By contrast, incidence of adipose tissue necrosis in the pancreas ranging up to 42% has been reported in fattening pigs [240]; the finding of chronic pancreatitis is made in these animals with commensurate frequency. This may be likened morphologically to the finding of lipolytic-proteolytic pancreatitis in man. In the course of our extensive animal studies we have seen disseminated adipose tissue necrosis in 4% of obese mongrel dogs (among 400 animals 5–15 years old) [476].

In evaluating experimental data [471], it is thus absolutely necessary to consider the physiological and pathoanatomical "baseline status" of the chosen exprimental animal in order to protect the investigator against misinterpretation of his observations and false inferences from analogy.

A comparison of human papillary forms "capable of pancreatitis" with those of species in which spontaneous pancreatitis has been reported [100] shows that the anatomical structure of the papilla itself cannot be of fundamental significance as far as the development of pancreatitis is concerned. On the other hand, the distal segment of the common bile duct often runs a partly intrapancreatic course in the dorsal head region; in this segment, accessory pancreatic duct openings are detectable in up to 80% of cases [85, 355] so that in the presence of a papillary concrement or papillary stenosis reflux is possible even without a common channel (incidence of impacted papillary stones approximately 1–3%; biliary reflux pancreatitis approximately 6%). This finding, moreover, can help explain the relatively high incidence of isolated head pancreatitis within the context of "cholecystopancreatitis" in human pathology. There is also evidence from animals pointing to a viral causation of individual cases of acute pancreatitis; during an epidemic in Canada up to 75% of the trout stock died of acute pancreatitis [469]; there have also been individual observations in dogs and rodents mainly involving coxsackievirus infections.

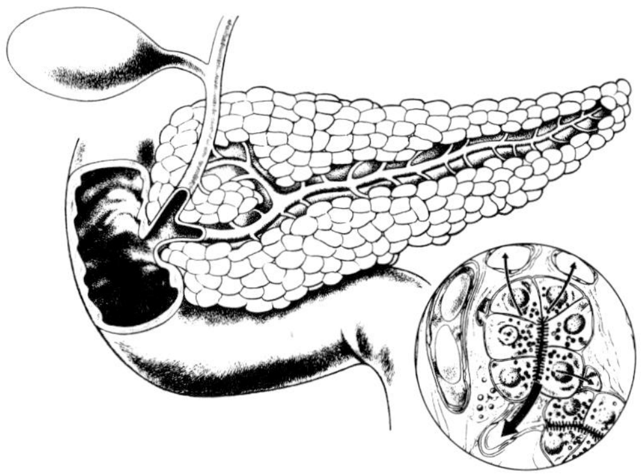

Fig. 8. Normal findings. Topographic relations between gallbladder, extrahepatic bile ducts, pancreas, and duodenum; papillary region with common channel and intrapancreatic course of common bile duct with accessory pancreatic ducts. (circle) histological detail (see caption of Fig. 19): main stream of secretions draining via ducts and secondary stream of secretions draining lymphogenously.

4.3   Biliary pancreatitis (BP)

Characteristics are: hemorrhagic-necrotizing biliary, primarily nonautodigestive acute pancreatitis; reflux pancreatitis as understood by Opie and Halsted with impacted papillary stone and common channel; acute biliary head pancreatitis with openings of accessory pancreatic ducts into retropancreatic and intrapancreatic segments of common bile duct in the presence of ductal concrements and no common channel.

This is the group of acute pancreatitides of canalicular origin which has frustrated previous efforts to reconcile etiology, pathogenesis, and morphogenesis and has thus cast doubt on the validity of collective surveys. Aside from the broad spectrum of pathophysiological and pathoanatomical data on the papillary and ductal regions (choledochous duct, duct of Wirsung, duct of Santorini; accessory pancreatic duct openings into the bile duct; presence or absence of a papilla minor) and their interrelations, it is the numerous precursory, accessory and associated diseases–take, for example, "pseudobiliary, cholecysto- and postoperative pancreatitis"–which are so variably evaluated regarding their pathogenetic significance (see Chapter 2).

BP begins with coagulation necrosis of pancreatic duct epithelia and of acini affected by reflux, disturbed circulation in the intra- and periductular vascular plexus, and vascular edema (in contrast to the primary dyschylous juice edema in LPP) and progresses in later stages to secondary autodigestion due to hypoxia and acidosis, with pancreatic juice edema and enzyme derangement.

With an impacted papillary stone and massive reflux, the full-blown picture of this disease form, as a pancreatic apoplexy, always corresponds to Kümmerle's severity stage III [258, 259] with a mortality rate ranging up to 100 % (Fig. 13, Plate II; Fig. 14, Plate III).

The morphological pattern and intraorganic distribution pattern of biliary reflux pancreatitis are determined by the amount of reflux, the substrate contact time, the prevailing concentration of unconjugated bile acids [447, 448], and the duct anatomy: Of prime importance are the interrelations between the common bile duct and the major or minor pancreatic duct plus the minor papilla as well as the presence or absence of accessory pancreatic *duct openings* into the common bile duct along its prepapillary retro- and intrapancreatic course (see Chapter 2).

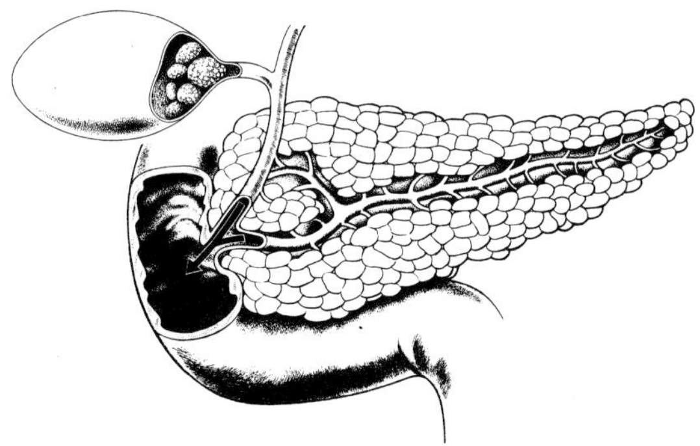

Fig. 9. Cholecystolithiasis may occur in combination with acute pancreatitis, as in Figs. 28, 29, 30, 32.

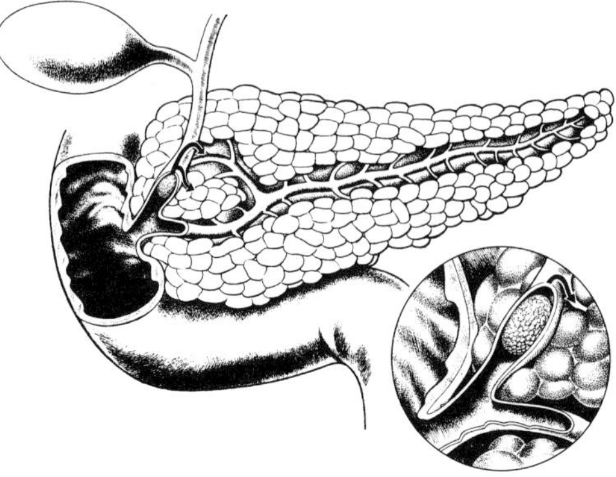

Fig. 10. Choledocholithiasis in presence of accessory pancreatic ducts; e.g., acute head pancreatitis as in Fig. 33. In circle, detail of duct, reflux pathway.

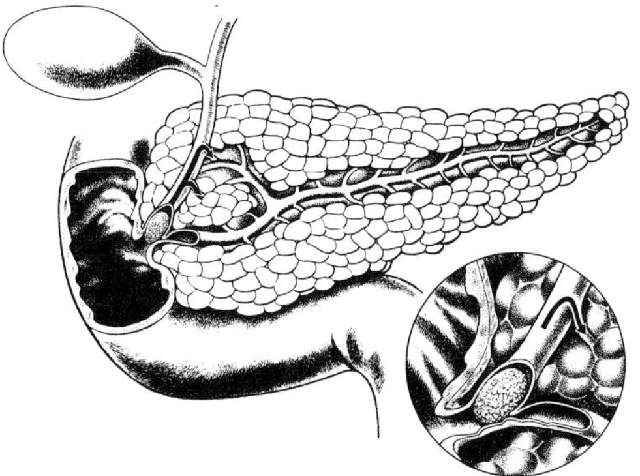

Fig. 11. Papillary concrements with compression of duct of Wirsung. Reflux possible via accessory pancreatic ducts, e.g., head pancreatitis as in Fig. 33.

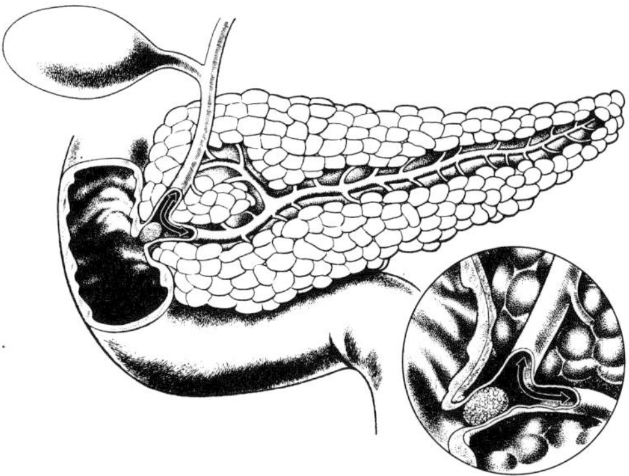

Fig. 12. Papillary concrements in presence of common channel, massive bile reflux. Pancreatic apoplexy, Opie type grade III, according to Kümmerle, Fig. 31. In circle, detail of bile reflux.

This anatomical "predestination" thus helps decide whether the process can be confined to the pancreatic head or involves the whole organ. If a major and a minor papilla exist and the two ductal systems communicate with one another, the duct of Santorini can function as an "overflow valve" despite impaction of a stone in the region of the papilla of Vater. In such cases the stone impaction will be associated only with transitory edema in the area of the pancreatic head but the full-blown picture of hemorrhagic necrosis will not develop. Analogous findings have been made in experimental pancreatitis of the dog if, following intraductular instillation of the noxa and ensuing duct ligation, no account is taken of the fact that the dog pancreas generally has two (in 84%) [469] but a maximum of four excretory ducts so that the infused material can flow back into the duodenum via anastomoses despite the duct ligation (Fig. 15, Plate III; Figs. 16–18, Plate IV).

The effect of sodium taurocholate administered to dogs or rats* as a 1–5% solution by intraductular instillation is comparable to that of the detergent Triton X–100. Coagulation necrosis results immediately after contact of the infusate with the pancreatic duct epithelia; if, upon application of high pressure, the infusate reaches the acini (as in the parenchymal phase in ERCP!), the acinar epithelia will also undergo coagulation necrosis (note and see also discussion of complications in ERCP, page 83). The intramural vascular network of the pancreatic ducts is strikingly hyperemic; rubrostasis and perirubrostasis are followed by massive erythrocyte diapedesis. Vascular edema and area hemorrhages cause primarily mechanical structural disruptions of the lobules and acini. The hypoxic acinar epithelia undergo vacuolar degeneration. The acinar epithelia are destroyed; there is no autodigestion primarily. The extent of the "chemical" pancreatic necrosis is correlated with the concentration, quantity, and contact time of the noxious agent; it can lead within less than 60 minutes to the full-blown picture of hemorrhagic pancreatitis with concurrent secretion against an obstacle (duct ligatures after instillation of noxa) and failure of intramural lymph circulation [469, 471, 488]. The hypoxic phase of biliary pancreatitis is additionally associated with activation of lipolytic and proteolytic proenzymes and a subsequent chain reaction. The acinar epithelial cells with their damaged membranes as well as the intrapancreatic and peripancreatic fat cells fall victim to lipolysis and proteolysis. Primary vascular and secondary juice edema produce additive effects following lymph blockade and intraorganic accumulation of enzymes. By the same token, acini that were not initially affected by the bile reflux now become involved in the "secondary" autodigestion by the "mixed" edema including the activated enzymes.

The *factor of time* is thus decisive for evaluation of the morphogenesis of biliary pancreatitis. The hemorrhagic component can complicate any form of pancreatitis in its late phase but it is especially characteristic of the biliary variant, predominating even in its initial stage.

In addition to the bile-induced vascular damage in biliary pancreatitis, there is an early increase in vascular permeability (capillary leak) of the histamine type, the pancreas being rich in mast cells and a shock organ [470, 491]. Generally speaking, therefore, the vascular factor may be of biliary, lipolytic, or proteolytic origin; it thus has multiple pathogenetic connotations.

---

* With regard to rat experiments, it should be borne in mind that these animals have no centroacinar cells, therefore the phenomenon of "isthmic blockade" known in human pathology cannot be produced in this species.

Table 6. Factors of pathogenetic importance for coincidence of biliary tract diseases and pancreatitis (see Chapter 2.4)

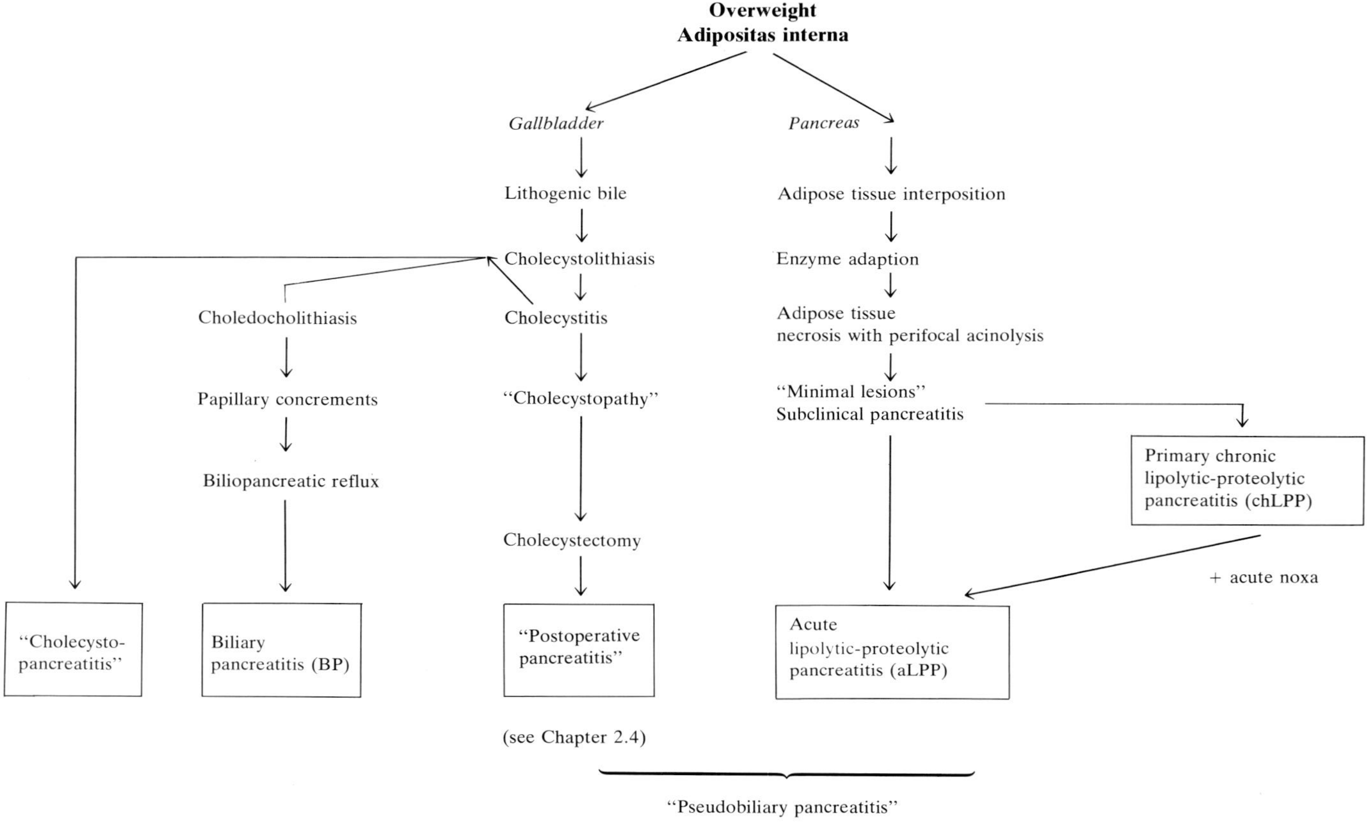

4.4   Mixed forms of acute pancreatitis (M. P.): Chyme reflux pancreatitis

The refluxing duodenal contents are a mixture of bile, chyme, and activated pancreatic enzymes. If the intracellularly stored fat in acinar dyschylia due to metabolic or hypoxic factors (see page 44) becomes the primary substrate of the – active – lipase and the focus of the lipolytic-proteolytic pancreatitis (LPP), chyme reflux carries the substrate to the lipase via the ductal system. The effect of emulsified fats on the pancreas following intraductular administration (instillation of olive oil with or without bile) had already been known to Claude Bernard in 1856. The effects of three components accumulate during chyme reflux:
1. bile,
2. substrate,
   plus
3. active or activated pancreatic enzymes.

The factors of decisive pathogenetic significance for the course, type, and severity of reflux pancreatitis are listed in Tables 7 and 8.

Table 7. Factors determining the course, type, and severity of pancreatitis

---

1. Composition of reflux
   (a) Duodenal contents, high/low fat content
       Duodenal contents, finely/coarsely emulsified
   (b) Content of active proteolytic and lipolytic enzymes
   (c) Ratio of conjugated to unconjugated bile acids
   (d) Bile plus duodenal contents with active lipolytic and proteolytic enzymes
2. Amount of reflux
3. Contact time
4. Causes of reflux
   (a) Papillary concrements
   (b) Papillary spasm
   (c) Papillary edema
   (d) Parasites in papillary-ductal system
   (e) Afferent loop syndrome following Billroth II gastric resection

---

Table 8. Pathogenesis and morphogenesis – secretion against an obstacle

---

Duct occlusions due to:
1. Edema of papilla of Vater related to general edema of duodenal mucosa
2. Pancreatolithiasis, concrements in ducts of Wirsung and Santorini
3. Metaplasia of duct epithelium, papillary folding/hyperplasia of duct epithelium
4. Cicatricial stenoses of pancreatic ducts
5. Choledocholithiasis, papillary lithiasis
6. Stenosing inflammation of papilla of Vater
7. Juxtapapillary duodenal diverticulum
8. Papillary carcinoma
9. Parasites (e.g., ductular ascension of ascarids)

Pathogenetically and morphogenetically, then, chyme reflux pancreatitis takes up an intermediate position between the hemorrhagic-necrotizing biliary form (BP) and the lipolytic-proteolytic-autodigestive form (LPP). Even in its early stages, one finds concurrent coagulation necroses of pancreatic duct and acinar epithelia as well as autodigestive parenchymal and mesenchymal necroses. The incidence of this form of pancreatitis amounts to approximately 10% of all cases of acute pancreatitis [480]; its severity in most cases conforms to stages II/III according to Kümmerle and Hollender at a mortality rate of about 80% [259]. From the outset, bile, substrate, and activated or active enzymes mark the morphogenesis of reflux pancreatitis; in individual cases it may prove very difficult to distinguish this form of pancreatitis from a primary LPP if the reflux that occurred and its causes can be verified neither diagnostically/operatively nor autopsically (particularly if the reflux was of short duration) and if the morphological alterations of the pancreatic duct epithelia and the intraductular and periductular vascular plexus are not very pronounced.

4.5 Lipolytic-proteolytic-autodigestive pancreatitis (LPP)

4.5.1 Morphological premises and phenomena
(Fig. 19, Plate V)

Acini are grouped around interposed fat cells or adjoin them subcapsularly. Physiological drainage of the pancreatic juice takes place mainly via the excretory duct system but also by parapedesis as accessory secretion passing between the acinar epithelia through the common basement membrane of an acinus into the interstitium [474], from which it is transported by the lymph. In man, the pancreatic ducts begin in the acinar lumen; their epithelia that extend into the acini are called centroacinar cells (= isthmic epithelial cells). The secretion is therefore passed primarily between the centroacinar cells (= isthmic epithelial cells) into the acinar lumen and via connecting ductules into intralobular excretory ducts. The term "isthmic epithelial cells" characterizes the physiological, hence also pathophysiological, import of this region more aptly than the anatomical name "centroacinar cells." In man, it is here, in the isthmus of the connecting ductules, that we find the anatomicohistologically given Achilles heel of pancreatic secretion with the danger of "isthmic blockade" [479], hence increase of parapedesis in the presence of "overload and functional decompensation" (see page 46). There is a dense capillary network in periacinar as well as intra- and periductular locations; this is supplied from the lobular periphery and also from postinsular capillaries; the latter thus contain blood already contaminated with hormones (insulin, glucagon) [118, 119, 451]: the "lobulo-insular unit" according to Thiel 1954. This vascular anatomy is significant for the balance between protective and aggressive factors (Table 8) in the induction of acute pancreatitis. A particularly large quantity of mast cells is found around vessels and acini in the interstitial tissue [145, 470, 491].

At the inception of LPP there is fat cell necrosis with perifocal acinolysis in the presence of adipositas interna or intrapancreatic adipose tissue proliferation [472, 475].

The incidence of such at first clinically silent lipolytic-proteolytic foci, or minimal lesions, increases from decade to decade in a lifetime and is significantly correlated with the quantity of intrapancreatic and peripancreatic adipose tissue (Tables 10, 11).

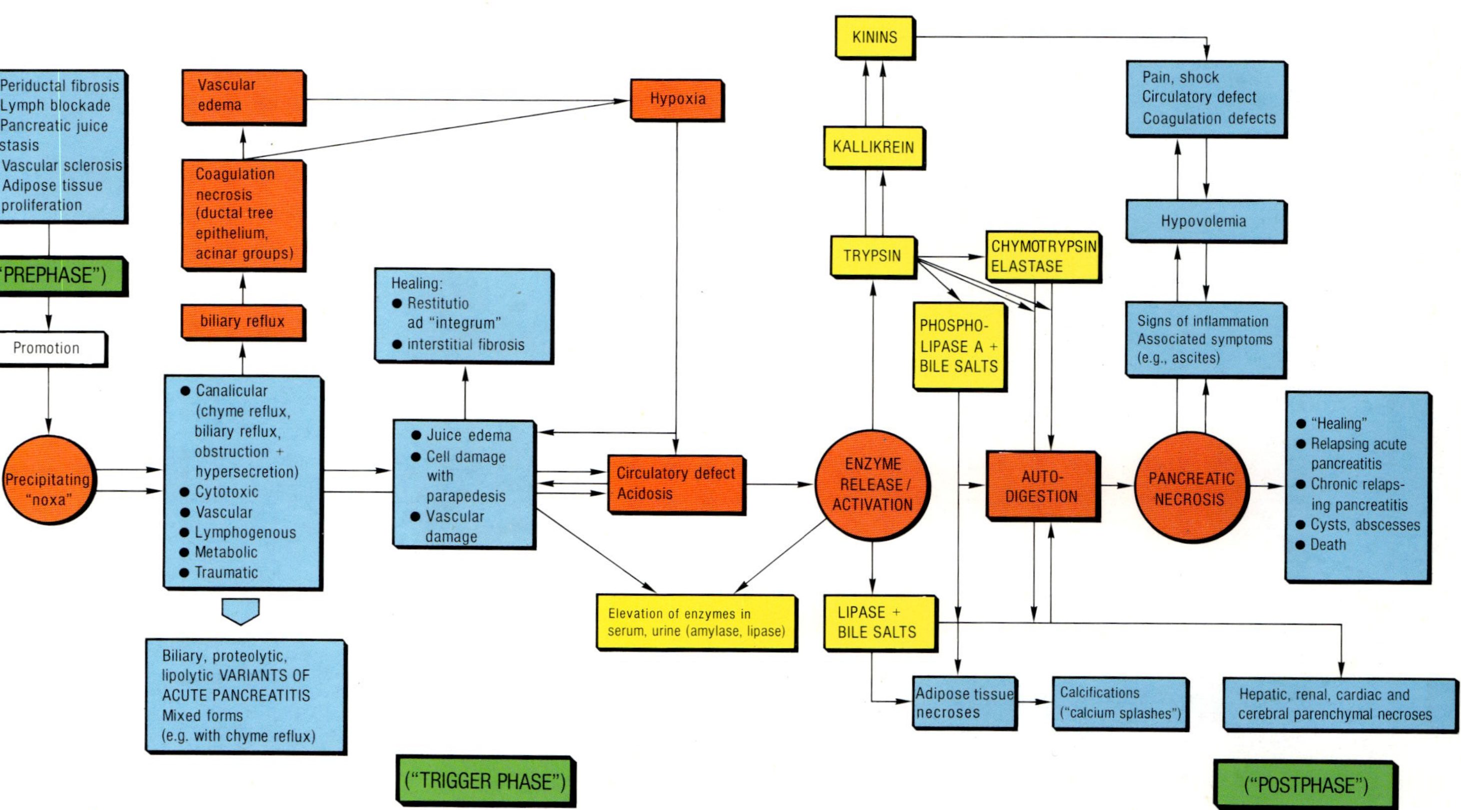

Fig. 4. Pathogenesis of acute pancreatitis (from Forell and Lehnert [128] and Wanke [478]).

Plate I

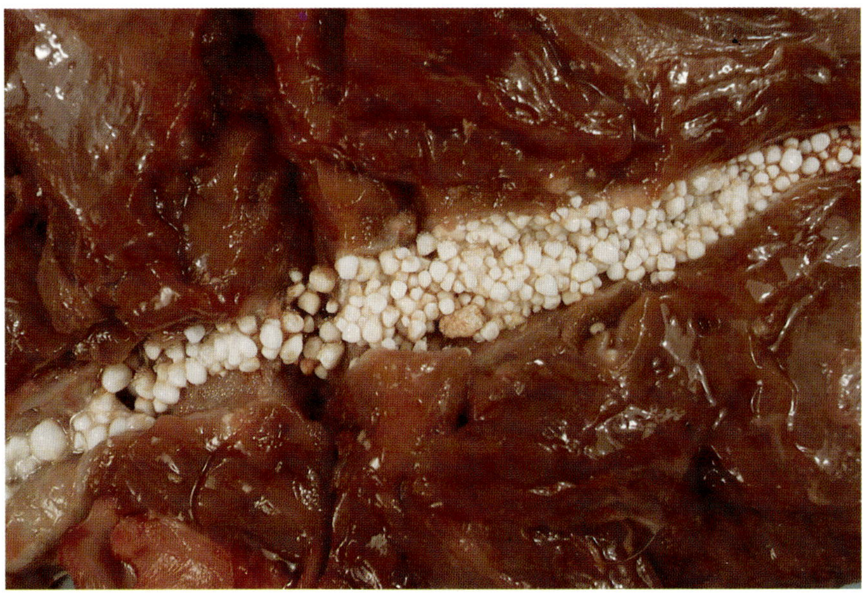

Fig. 7. Bovine pancreas; marked sialolithiasis; despite secretion against obstacle, no pancreatitis since bovine pancreas produces only traces of lipase and there is no substrate for initial lipolysis.

Fig. 13. Pancreatic apoplexy in presence of common channel; papillary stone and biliopancreatic reflux; female, age 64.

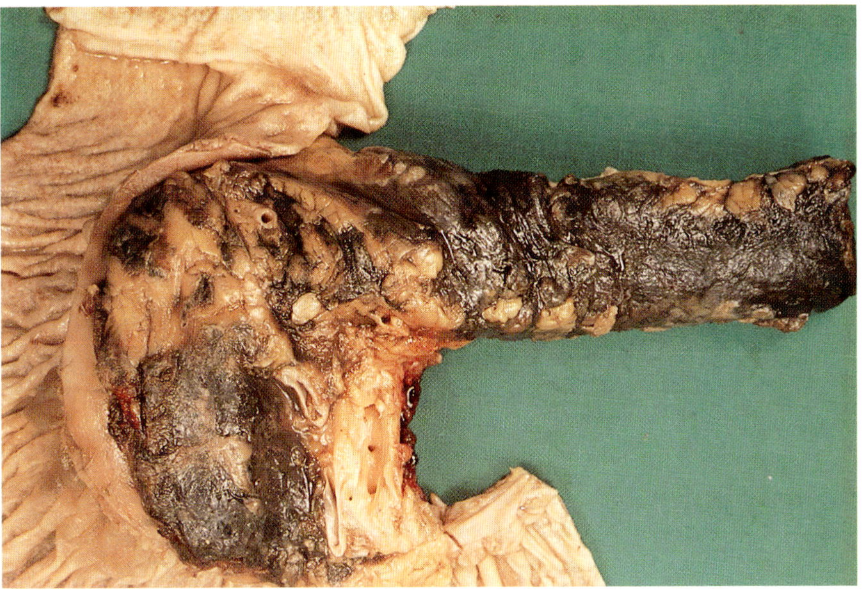

Plate II

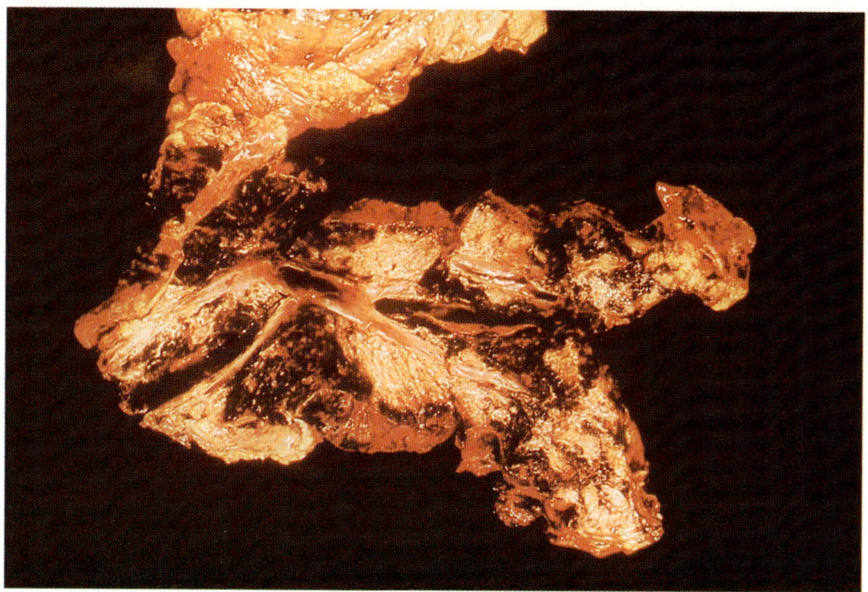

Fig. 14. Incomplete pancreatic apoplexy; hemorrhagic-necrotizing pancreatitis with biliopancreatic reflux; female, age 59.

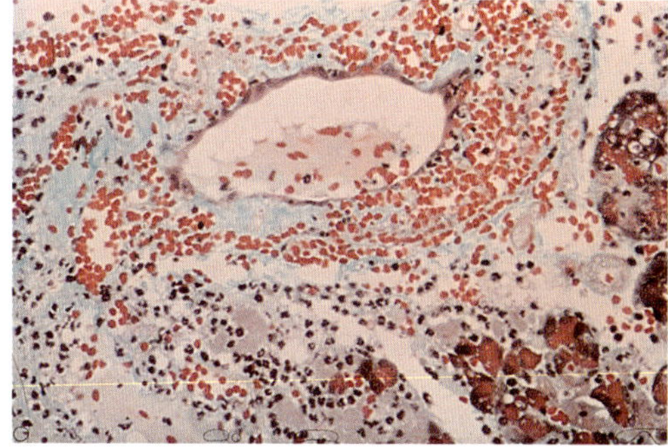

Fig. 15. Biliary pancreatitis; after bile reflux, due to detergent effect, necrosis of pancreatic duct epithelia, hemorrhages, and coagulation necrosis of acinar cell complexes affected by reflux.

Plate III

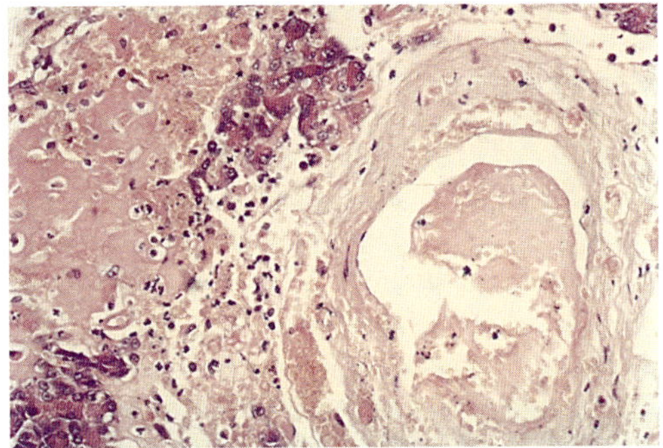

Fig. 16. Biliary pancreatitis. Subtotal coagulation necrosis of a pancreatic duct and perifocal acini.

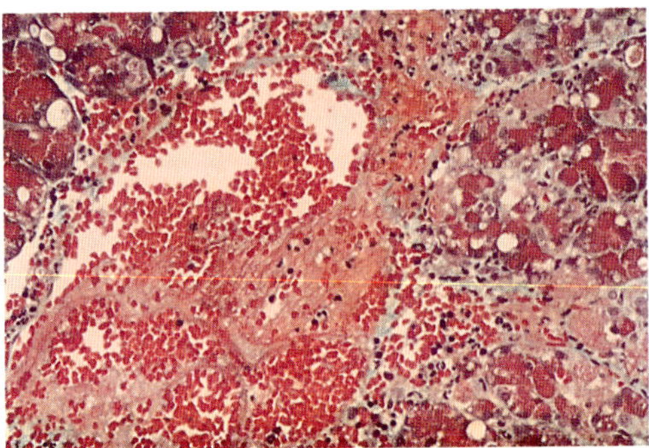

Fig. 17. Biliary pancreatitis. Hemorrhagic-vascular edema with mechanical rupture of lobular and acinar structural cohesion; hypoxic damage.

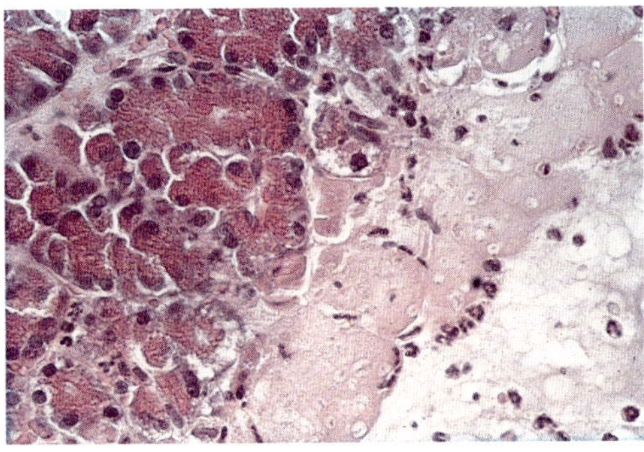

Fig. 18. Late phase of biliary pancreatitis: in hypoxia, secondary dyschylous pancreatic juice edema with autodigestive acinar necrosis associated with enzyme-rich juice edema.

Plate IV

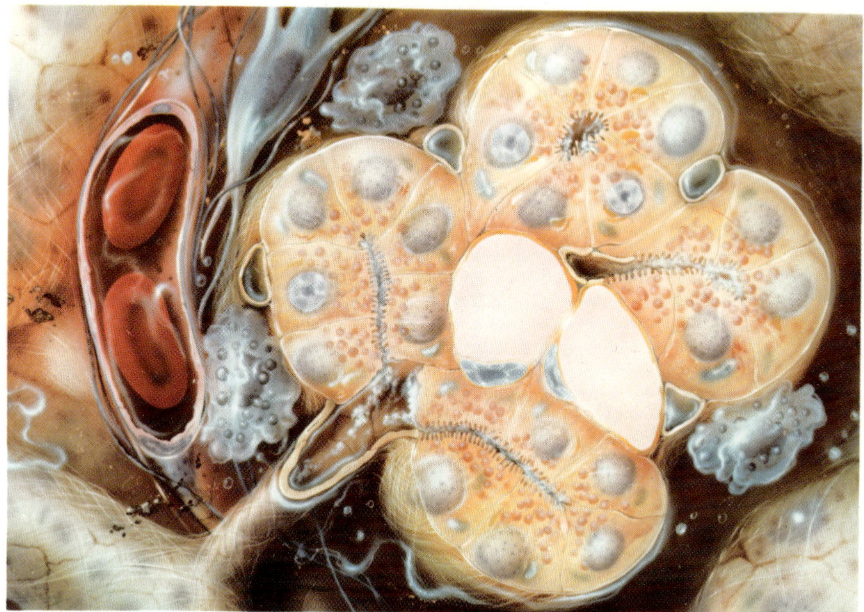

Fig. 19. Morphological premises of autodigestive lipolytic-proteolytic pancreatitis. Four acini with their epithelia are grouped around two centrally situated fat cells; physiological drainage of pancreatic juice passes through initial pancreatic ducts bordered by isthmic epithelial cells into larger excretory ducts. Accessory secretions pass via the common cell basis of the acinar epithelia (by parapedesis) into the interstitium and drain primarily via lymph vessels. An abundant capillary plexus ensures optimal oxygen supply. In interstitial tissue, mast cells are around vessels and acini; the pancreas is an organ rich in mast cells. In perivascular space, are collagenous and elastic fibers as well as fibrocytes.

Plate V

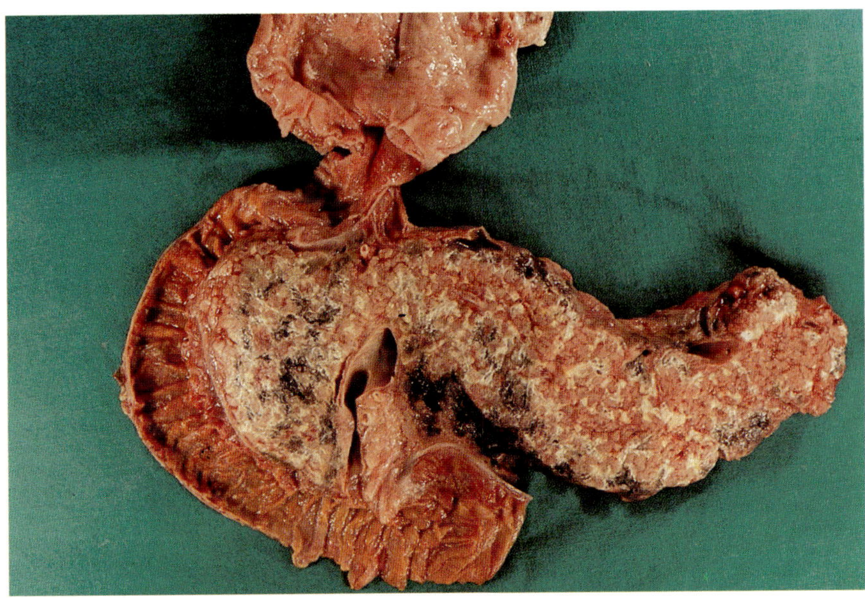

Fig. 20. Lipolytic-proteolytic pancreatitis; female, age 78.

Fig. 21. Adipositas interna, general arteriosclerosis, diabetes mellitus; extensive areas of lipolytic-proteolytic necrosis involving the entire organ, with incipient hemorrhages.

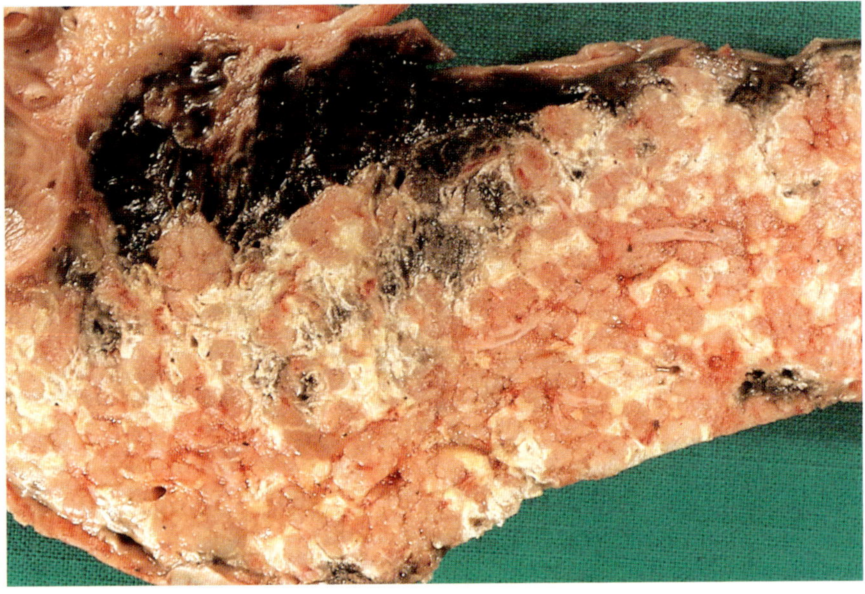

Plate VI

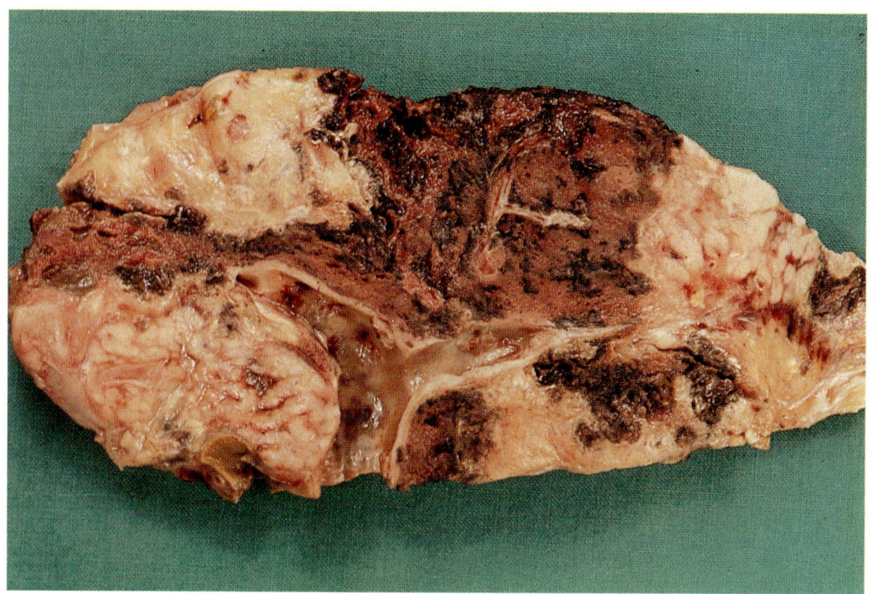

Fig. 22. Lipolytic-proteolytic pancreatitis: female, age 74.

Fig. 23. Obesity, senile emphysema, chronic cor pulmonale; segmental necrosis of markedly hemorrhagic character; incipient venous thrombosis, splenic vein.

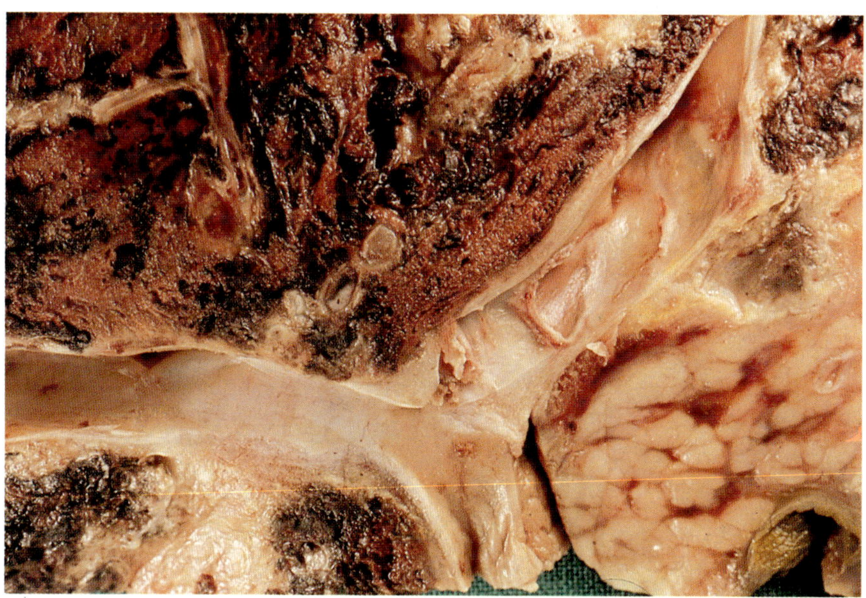

Plate VII

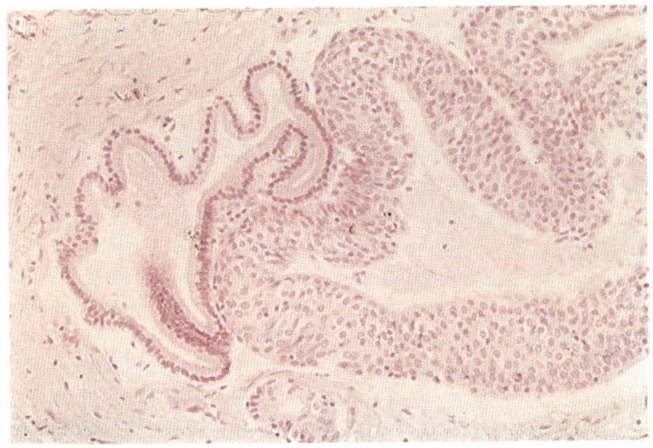

Precursory phase of acute pancreatitis.

Fig. 24. Squamous metaplasia of pancreatic duct epithelia.

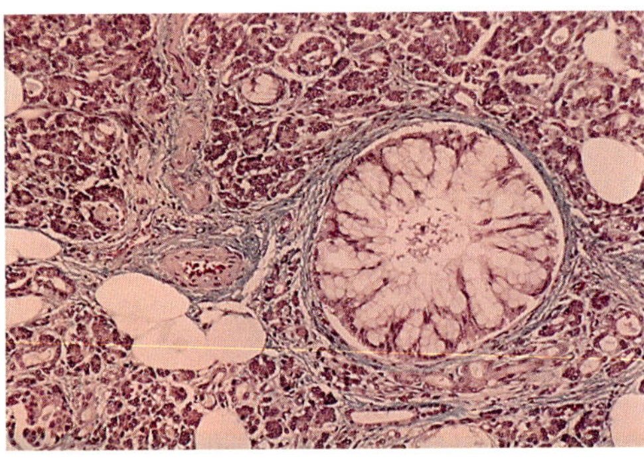

Fig. 25. Papillary hyperplasia of pancreatic duct epithelia with severe constriction of ductal lumen; incipient adipose tissue proliferation in vacated spaces with disseminated dyschylous atrophy.

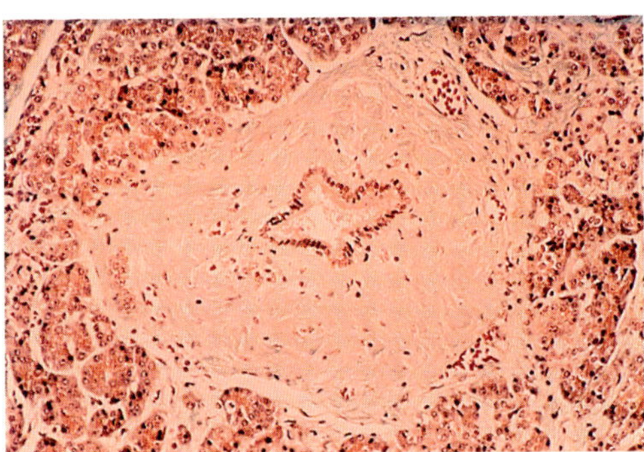

Fig. 26. Periductular fibrosis with lymphatic channel sclerosis.

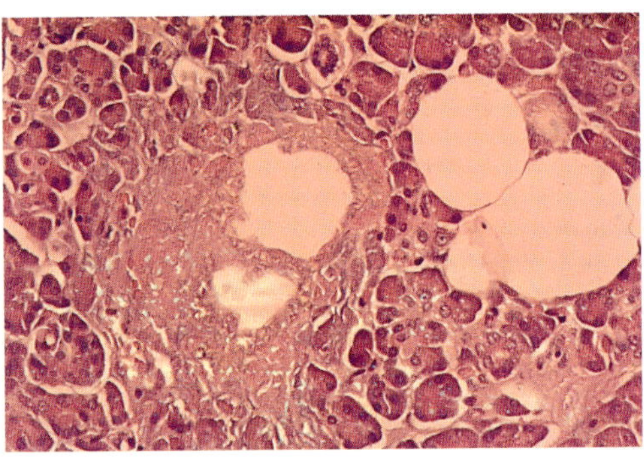

Fig. 27. Proliferation of adipose tissue in vacated spaces; lipolytic-proteolytic minimal lesions.

Plate VIII

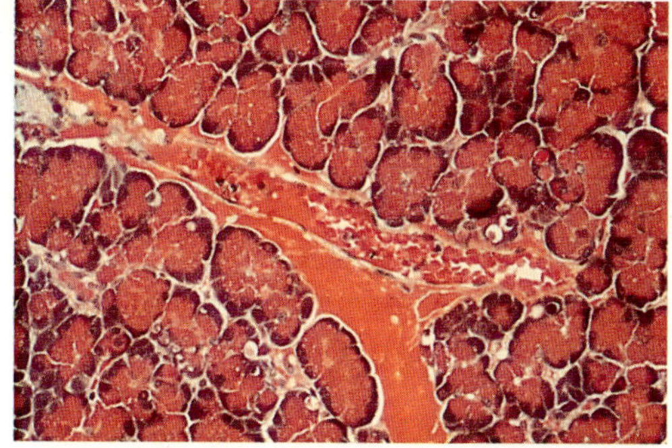

"Edematous pancreatitis".

Fig. 35. Circulatory defect, interstitial vascular edema. (a) Early stage.

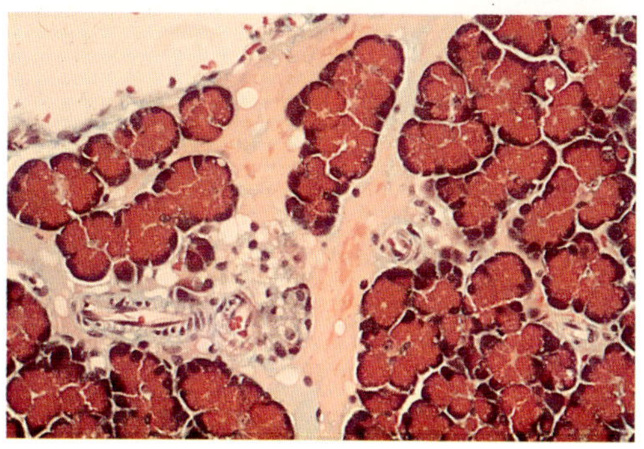

Fig. 36. (b) Late stage.

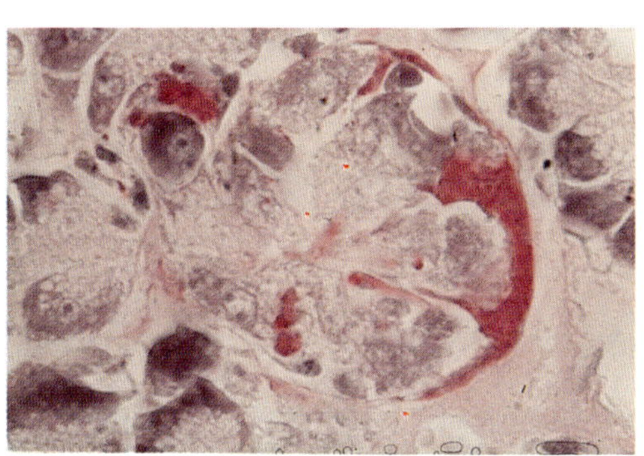

Fig. 37. Dyschylous pancreatic juice edema; (a) Early stage.

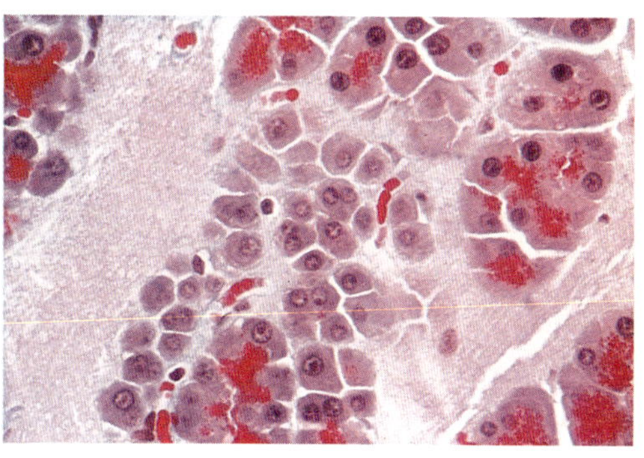

Fig. 38. (b) Late stage.

Plate IX

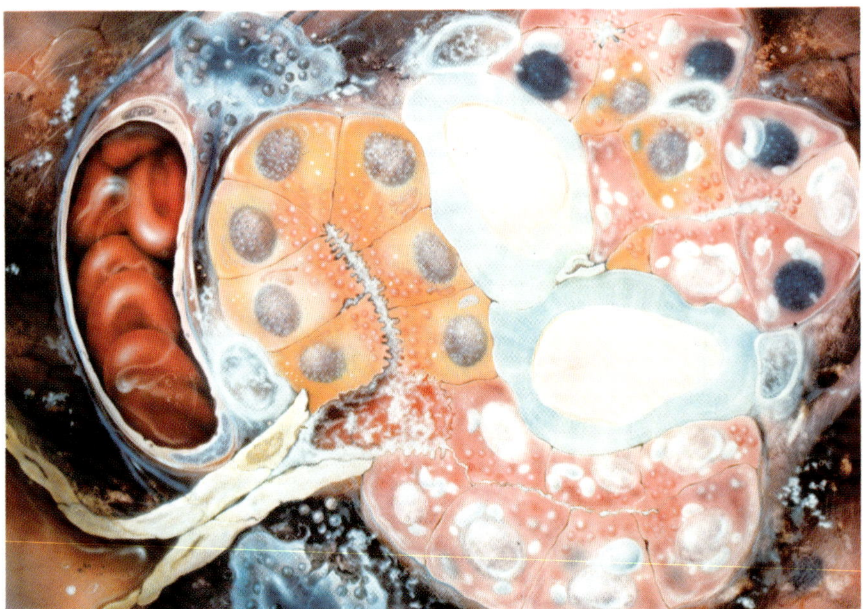

Fig. 39. *Early phase* of autodigestive lipolytic-proteolytic pancreatitis, semischematic.

This begins with fat cell necrosis. Two central interacinar areas of fat cell necrosis; owing to triglyceride cleavage and local acidosis activation of lipolytic and proteolytic proenzymes in perifocal acinar complexes with autodigestion. Four acini with their epithelia in various stages of cellular necrosis, such as eosinophil degeneration, nuclear pyknosis, karyorrhexis, karyolysis, 1 + 2 = target cell phenomenon = minimal lesion. The isthmic epithelia, also affected by hypoxia, undergo disordered hydration and swell up. Occlusion of initial ductules = isthmic blockade. The juice can no longer drain canalicularly and enters the interstitial tissue exclusively via parapedesis (increased parapedesis). Dyschylous juice edema with systemic enzymatic derangement. Up to these changes *(1–4)* the pancreatitis remains "edematous" and there is a possibility of compensation provided that there is adequate lymph drainage and inhibitor capacity.
If the number of minimal lesions increases, the lymph channels are plugged by the afflux of juice and cell debris = lymph blockage. Changes 1–4 are accompanied by mast cell degranulation with release of mesenchymal enzymes and decompensation of preterminal and terminal vasculature. The autodigestion thus spreads to the interstitium, involving collagenous and elastic fibers, the interstitial tissue and the vessels.

Plate X

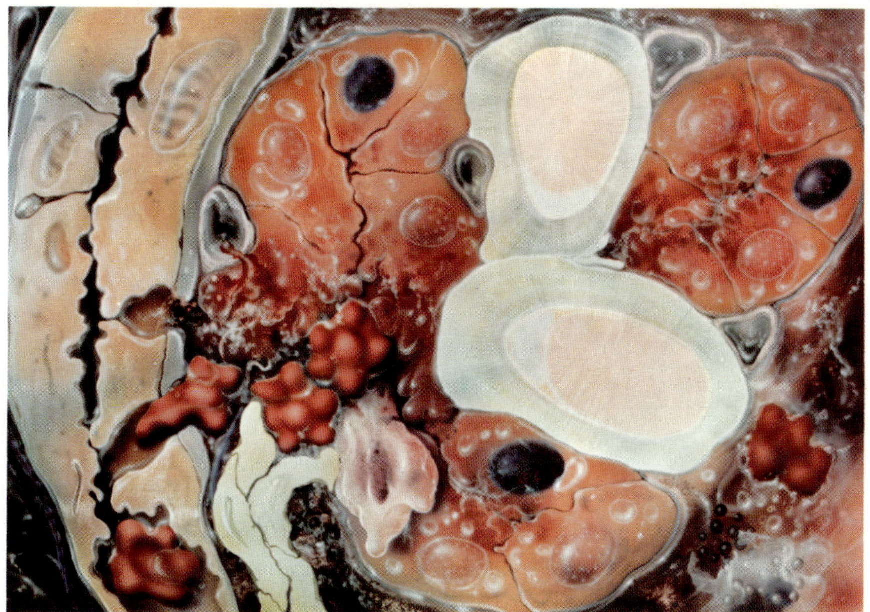

Fig. 40. *Late phase* of autodigestive lipolytic-proteolytic pancreatitis, semischematic.

The full-blown picture of acute autodigestive pancreatitis is marked by adipose tissue necrosis, pancreatic juice edema, parenchymal necrosis, and hemorrhages. In the individual case, the prognosis depends on the extent of the necrotic-autodigestive process and the "mixture ratio" of the four components.
Grouped around two central areas of fat cell necrosis with saponification are necrobiotic acini in varying stages of epithelial necrosis. Dyschylous juice edema of high enzyme and protein content fills the interstitium owing to isthmic blockade and lymph blockage. Rupture and degranulation of tissue mast cells and capillary wall edema with capillary leak in acidosis produce incompetence of preterminal and terminal vasculature with erythrocyte diapedesis and hemorrhagic edema. Widening of the transit zone closes the vicious cycle.

Plate XI

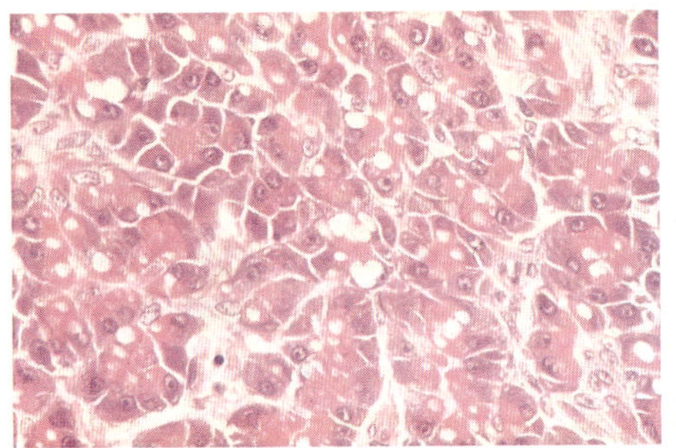

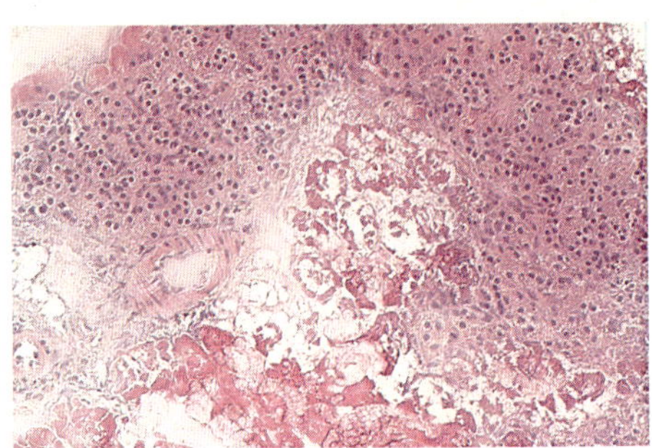

Fig. 41.   Fig. 45.

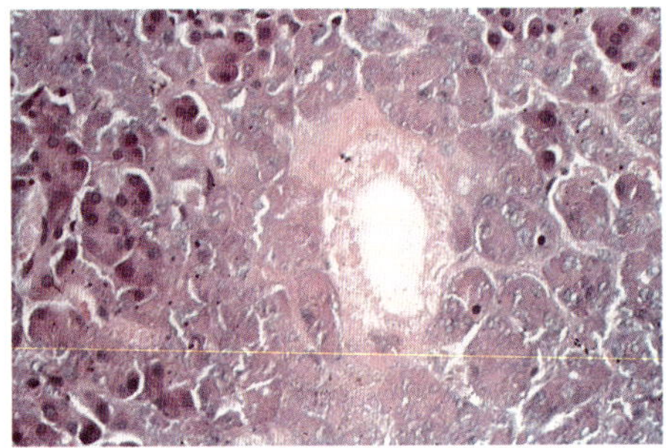

Fig. 42.

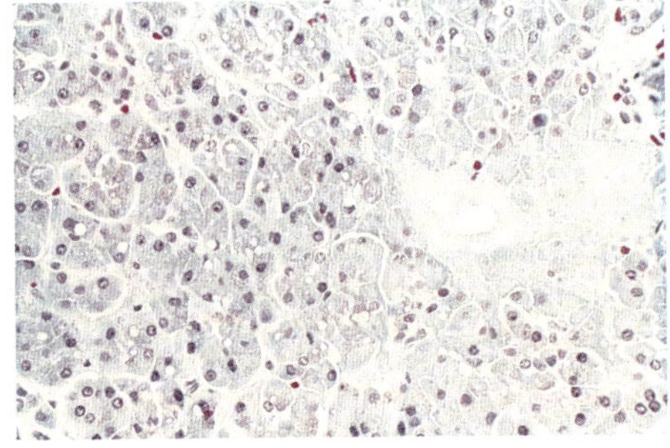

Fig. 43.

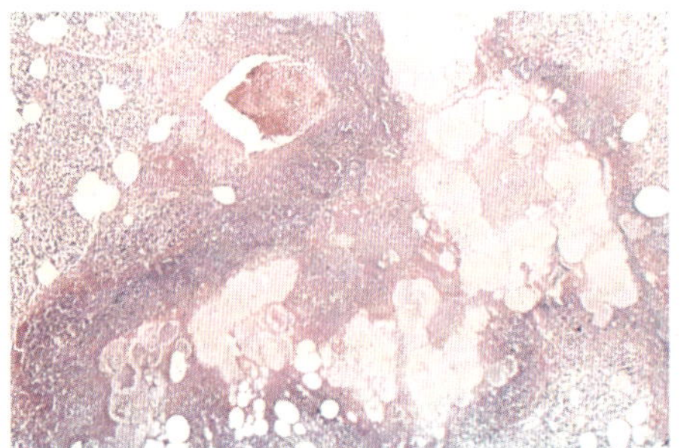

Fig. 44.

Plate XII

Autodigestion:

Fig. 41. Juxtanuclear hypoxic vacuolation of acinar epithelium. Male, age 25, hypovolemic shock, generalized acidosis.

Fig. 42. Early stage of lipolytic-proteolytic pancreatitis. "Target cell phenomenon": central fat cell necrosis, perifocal acinolysis with karyorrhexis and karyolysis. Male, age 10, hypovolemic shock.

Fig. 43. Same as Fig. 42 plus hypoxic vacuolation of acinar epithelium.

Fig. 44. Late stage of lipolytic-proteolytic pancreatitis with extensive proteolytic necrosis around areas of lipolytic necrosis in adipositas interna with incipient thrombosis. Female, age 78, adipositas interna, diabetes mellitus, generalized arteriosclerosis.

Fig. 45. Proteolytic digestion histotopochemically demonstrable above fresh areas of autodigestive necrosis by the method of "fibrinolysis autographs" (Todd 1959).

Table 9a. Pathogenetic-morphogenetic synopsis of acute pancreatitis

Prephase

Morphological

Humoral

(a) Intra-/peripancreatic
     adipose tissue proliferation
     Adipositas interna
(b) Vascular sclerosis
(c) Lymph blockage
     1. intramural, e.g., in
        periductular and
        periacinar fibrosis
     2. extramural, e.g., in
        obstruction of cysterna chyli
(d) Pancreatic juice stasis
     1. Squamous epithelial
        metaplasia or papillary
        hyperplasia of pancreatic
        duct epithelia
     2. Pancreatic duct stenoses
     3. Scaly dyschylia/lithiasis
     4. Stenosing inflammation of
        papilla of Vater or
        sclerosis of sphincter

(a) Enzyme adaptation
     1. Alimentary
        dys-/hyperproteinemia
        Hyperlipemia
     2. Hormonal,
        e.g., polyadenomatosis
(b) Secretory stimuli
     1. Alimentary
     2. Hormonal/neural
     3. "Toxic,"
        e.g., alcoholism, uremia

Focal energy insufficiency/acidosis/mechanical factors

Lipolytic-proteolytic "minimal lesions"
Subclinical pancreatitis

Tab. 9b. Pathogenetic-morphogenetic synopsis of acute pancreatitis

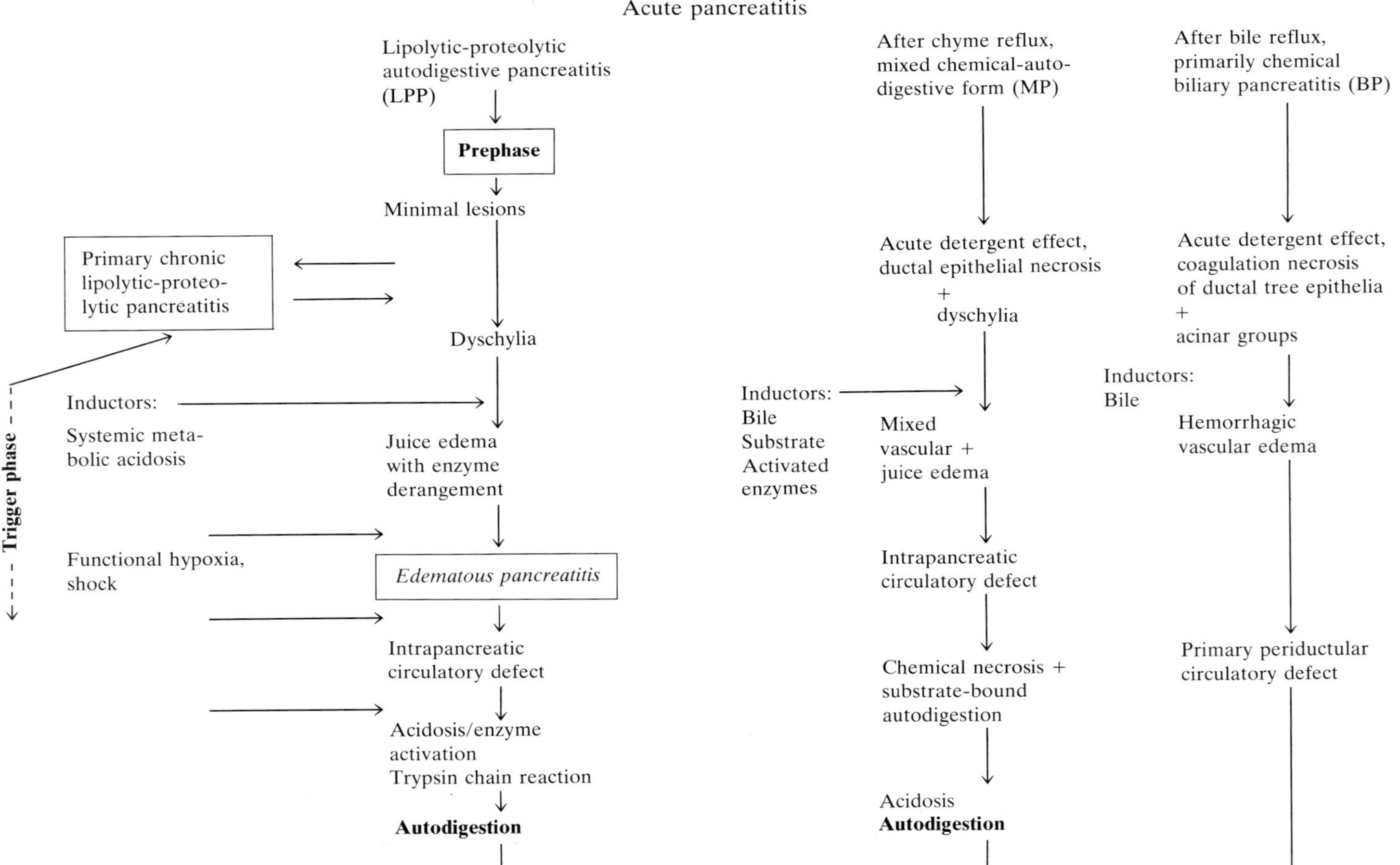

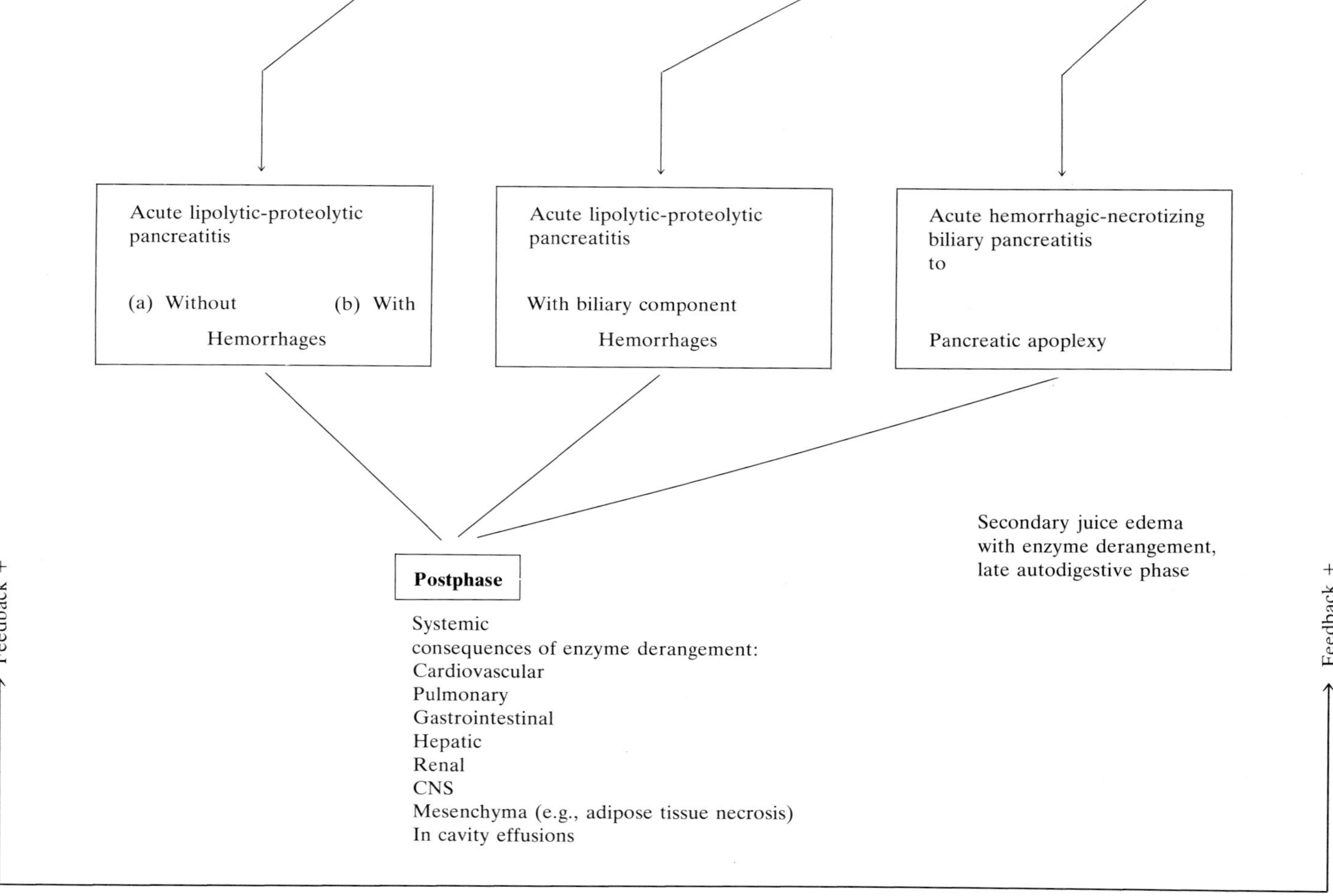

Acute lipolytic-proteolytic pancreatitis
(a) Without
(b) With
Hemorrhages
Acute lipolytic-proteolytic pancreatitis
With biliary component
Hemorrhages
Acute hemorrhagic-necrotizing biliary pancreatitis
to
Pancreatic apoplexy
Postphase
Systemic consequences of enzyme derangement:
Cardiovascular
Pulmonary
Gastrointestinal
Hepatic
Renal
CNS
Mesenchyma (e.g., adipose tissue necrosis)
In cavity effusions
Secondary juice edema with enzyme derangement, late autodigestive phase
Feedback +
Feedback +

Table 10. Relations between adipose tissue interposition, adipose tissue necrosis and perifocal acinolysis, based on 719 autopsies [475]

Adipose tissue interposition (%)	Adipose tissue necrosis (%)	Perifocal acinolysis (%)	Age (years)	No. of cases
5.6	5.4	4.5	1–15	354
14.3	6.9	6.9	16–25	245
62.7	34.6	31.0	+25	
			△58	120

Table 11. Body weights of 164 (94 male, 70 female) patients who died of acute pancreatitis

	Male	Female	Σ	
+	41	49	90 = 54.9%	+
NC	17	7	24 = 14.6%	NC
–	36	14	50 = 30.5%	–

+, overweight
NC, normal weight
–, underweight

Increase of the intrapancreatic adipose tissue is a common finding beyond age 50 (see discussion of risk factors and prognostic indices [372]), reportedly occurring to an appreciable degree in 60% [467] or 63% [475] of cases. This pancreatic transformation with lipolytic-proteolytic foci (minimal lesions) is accompanied by morphological changes which conform to the pattern of chronic pancreatitis en miniature and which, according to Wanke [472, 476], represent an important component of the precursory phase in about 85% of cases of acute pancreatitis (see below): the "unitary concept" of the origin of autodigestive, primarily nonbiliary pancreatitis [41, 100]. Considering the body weights of patients who died of acute pancreatitis (Tables 10, 11) the correlations between adipose tissue interposition/obesity/body weight and the severity and extent of LPP are of significance; only about 15% of those who died of aLPP, BP, or MP had normal weight, while the remainder showed adipose tissue interposition with obesity or adipose tissue proliferation and cachexia (Figs. 20, 21, Plate VI; Figs. 22, 23, Plate VII). Moreover, this adipositas interna of the pancreas is associated with commensurate frequency with extensive fatty infiltration of hepatic epithelia or fatty liver as defined by Kalk and with cholecystocholedocholithiasis (see also discussion of problems posed by so-called "cholecystopancreatitis" or "pseudobiliary pancreatitis").

Morphological findings in the prephase (Table 9a), besides adipose tissue interposition, include as a major risk factor periductular and interlobular fibrosis with lymph channel obliteration and recurrent juice edema as well as general and intraorganic vascular sclerosis. See also age distribution of acute pancreatitis (Table 1 and Table 12), comparison of underlying disease A vs. pathogenetic principle B, and the risk factor of "over age 50" as defined by Ranson.

Table 12. Acute and acute relapsing pancreatitis: 172 cases among 15,697 continuous autopsies of patients past 1 year of age who died (Heidelberg/Rendsburg 1963/1981)

A. Underlying disease		n
1. General arteriosclerosis		107 = 62%
2. Overweight (adipositas externa/interna)		94 = 55%
3. Heart and lung diseases		
(cardiosclerosis, chronic cor pulmonale, etc.)		83 = 48%
4. Liver and biliary tract diseases		74 = 43%
(a) Cholecystitis/		
Cholecystolithiasis	43	
(b) Cirrhosis of liver	27	
(c) Hepatitis	4	
5. Diabetes mellitus		50 = 29%
6. Gastroduodenal ulcers		38 = 22%
7. Postoperative		35 = 20%
8. Alcoholism		29 = 17%
9. Chronic renal insufficiency/uremia		21 = 12%
10. Malignant tumors		21 = 12%
11. Endocrinously active tumors or hyperplasia		6 = 3.5%
(a) Cushing's disease	3	
(b) Hyperparathyroidism	2	
(c) Hyperthyroidism	1	
12. Endocarditis		5 = 3%
13. Burns		2
14. E-605 intoxication		2

B. Pathogenetic principles
1. Vascular, hypoxic, acidosis
2. Metabolic
3. Vascular, hypoxic, acidosis, shock
4. Canalicular (biliary or chyme reflux pancreatitis), traumatic-iatrogenic (see Table 3, Postoperative pancreatitis), shock, e.g., peritoneal, metabolic (see Table 6, Pseudobiliary pancreatitis)
5. Vascular, acidosis, metabolic
6. Vascular, canalicular, traumatic-iatrogenic, metabolic "as common underlying factors"
7. See Table 3, Postoperative pancreatitis
8. Vascular, canalicular-dyschylous, metabolic-dysproteinemic (see Chapter 2)
9. Vascular, canalicular-dyschylous, metabolic-dysproteinemic, acidosis
10. Metabolic-dysproteinemic, canalicular-obstructive, vascular-old age, iatrogenic-postoperative
11. Metabolic-hormonal
12. Shock, acidosis
13. Dysproteinemic, shock
14. Hypoxic, shock

1–14:

Acidosis, dysproteinemia, obesity	38%
Biliary-pseudobiliary pancreatitis	25%
Postoperative pancreatitis	20%
Pancreatitis in alcoholism	17%

This prephase generally does not arise in children and young adults; accordingly, acute pancreatitis is encountered only in exceptional cases [429, 475, 483] and then has special etiological characteristics, being related, e.g., to malformations, trauma, hypoxia-acidosis-uremia, dyspepsia-burns-protein deficiency, polyadenomatosis, hyperlipoproteinemia, cirrhosis of the liver, or bacterial-viral infections.

Concurrently with the components of the prephase (Figs. 24–27, Plate VIII) involving the pancreas itself, liver and biliary tract diseases develop which often show no causal interrelations with the pancreatic changes ("pseudobiliary pancreatitis"–see diagram). This group includes the majority of so-called idiopathic pancreatitides and pancreatitis in alcohol abuse, hence the large group of "metabolically" induced disease cases. In alcoholics in particular, a phase of initially inhibited secretory output is followed by stimulation of enzyme secretion, increase of protein concentrations in the pancreatic juice with precipitation of protein plugs in the small pancreatic ducts [159, 162, 211, 283, 399, 401] and, with it, the phenomenon of scaly proteodyschylia with or without microlithiasis (see discussion of involvement of pancreas in uremia [478]), secretion against an obstacle, recurrent enzyme derangement, and danger of acute exacerbation, e.g., with increasing adipose tissue interposition (see Prephase).

The acute exacerbation of the lipolytic-proteolytic "minimal lesions" as the preparatory ground comes about:

(a) hematogenously through direct damage to the organelles of the anabolic and functional metabolism of the acinar epithelial cells in the metabolic form, e.g., in the context of alcohol abuse with proteodyschylia, as well as through damage to the organelles of cell respiration in hypoxia, acidosis and shock–the pancreas as a shock organ;
(b) lymphogenously via adjacent organs or metastatically;
(c) mesenchymally after liberation of mast cell enzymes (as in shock) and also by an indirect hematogenous route as a septic excretory inflammation–the pancreas as an excretory organ;
(d) ductally due to bile or chyme reflux or through bacterial-parasitic ascension.

The extent of organ destruction depends on the extent of the imbalance between aggressive and protective factors (Table 13), [28, 31, 41, 474]: hence on the extent of lipolytic-proteolytic necrosis and on the absence or presence of complicating vascular erosion; if this is present, especially when seen macroscopically during operation, the hemorrhagic component may come to the foreground–actually or seemingly–as a perifocal hyperemic reaction and prevent intraoperative differentiation from the classic biliary form (BP) as defined by Opie (Opie type). From this point of view one can un-

Table 13. Protective mechanisms against induction of acute pancreatitis

1. Continuous and unimpeded flow of pancreatic juice
2. Adequate mucous secretion of duct epithelium
3. Synthesis of proteolytic enzymes and phospholipases as inactive precursors, storage in zymogen granules
4. Supply of protease inhibitors in acinar cells, pancreatic secretion, and in serum
5. Concurrent secretion of enzymes and inhibitor
6. Directed permeability of acinar epithelia ("shoked parapedesis")
7. Inactivation of interstitially secreted (by parapedesis) juice
8. Lack of intrapancreatic substrate for lipolytic enzymes
9. Unobstructed lymph efflux
10. Sufficient blood flow through organ synchronous with secretion

derstand the rough clinical distinction between "edematous pancreatitis," on one hand, and "hemorrhagic-necrotizing pancreatitis," on the other hand, though this is risky from the pathoanatomical standpoint for prognostic-therapeutic assessment of the individual case.

On one hand, LPP is closely related to the edematous form; it develops in a disseminated, areal, pseudosegmental manner or as a total organ necrosis but it may then macroscopically appear hemorrhagic-necrotizing, assuming the severity of grades II to III according to Kümmerle and Hollender [258, 259, 415].

LPP of grade I remains clinically silent as a rule (minimal lesions) or changes into the "edematous form."

With respect to its morphogenesis, edematous pancreatitis, too, is predominantly a component of acute lipolytic-proteolytic pancreatitis, which progresses through the stages of

> dyschylia,
> edema,
> circulatory disorder,
> necrobiosis,
> and autodigestion.

The process can come to a halt at each stage. This is made clear by the definition of a prephase, which itself goes on to dyschylia, and also becomes manifest in the severity ratings derived from clinical experience. Grades I, II, and III thus correspond morphologically to:

I =	Edematous pancreatitis	Mild form
	(a) "Bland" biliary form	
	(b) Early stage of aLPP	
II =	Partially necrotizing pancreatitis	Moderately severe
	(a) "Bland" biliary form	form
	(b) Lipolytic-proteolytic form with or without low-grade hemorrhages	
III =	Diffusely necrotizing pancreatitis	Severe form
	(a) Biliary form–pancreatic apoplexy	
	(b) aLPP with diffusely hemorrhagic-necrotizing component	

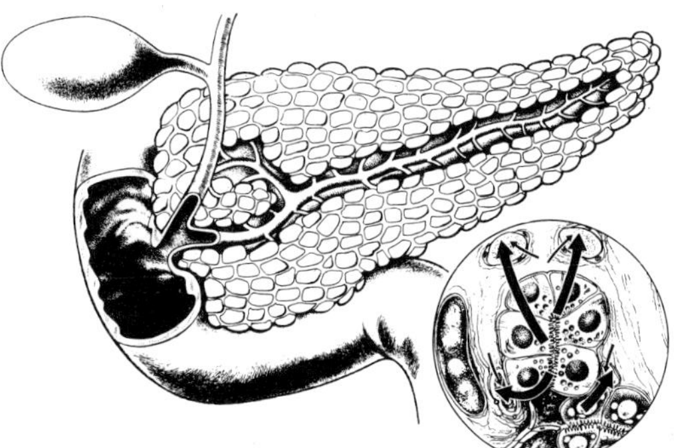

Fig. 28. Edematous pancreatitis, Kümmerle grade I. Organ enlarged (see CT findings); lobules spread apart by interstitial juice edema; no destruction. Histological detail in circle (see caption of Fig. 39): After isthmic blokkade, main secretion given off interstitially and draining lymphogenously = "compensated edema."

Fig. 29. Minimal lesions, subclinical lipolytic-proteolytic pancreatitis (LPP); reference points to chronic pancreatitis (chLPP); focal necrosis in adipositas interna with intra- and peripancreatic adipose tissue proliferation (into vacated spaces) or interposition. Histological detail in circle (see caption of Fig. 39): Target cell phenomena with disseminated acinar epithelial necrosis linked to adipose tissue necrosis; interstitial juice edema following focal isthmic blockade–still lymphogenously "compensated edema."

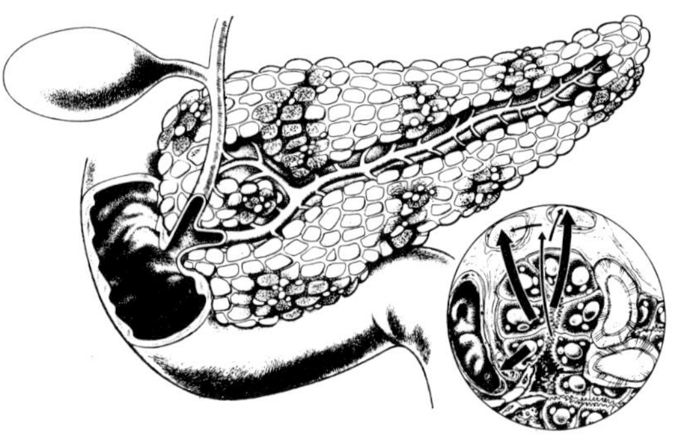

Fig. 30. Acute lipolytic-proteolytic segmental or focal pancreatitis (aLPP), Kümmerle grade II.
Minimal lesions with adipose tissue interposition and focally-segmentally confluent necrotic foci with/without hemorrhages. Histological detail in circle (see caption, Fig. 40): Advanced autodigestive lobular necrosis adjacent to areas of fat cell necrosis, isthmus blockade, incompetence of terminal vasculature, hemorrhages due to diapedesis and rupture; focal-segmental decompensated edema.

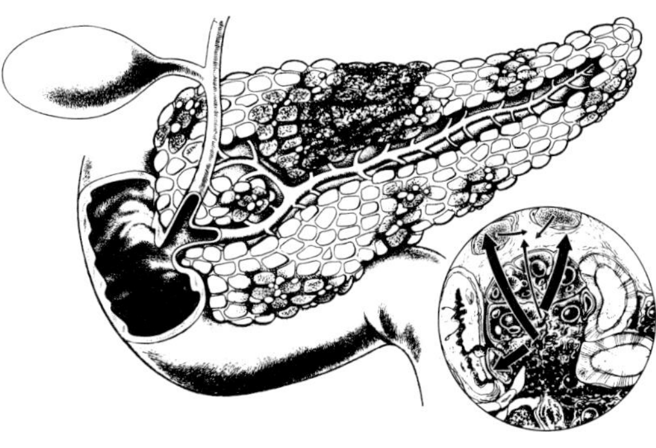

Fig. 31. Acute hemorrhagic-necrotizing pancreatitis, Kümmerle grade III.
Histological detail in circle (see caption, Fig. 40): Acinar necrosis, fat cell necrosis, hemorrhages, decompensated hemorrhagic edema.

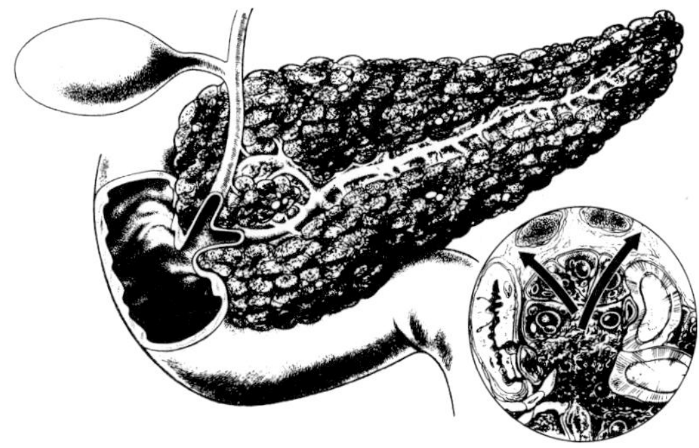

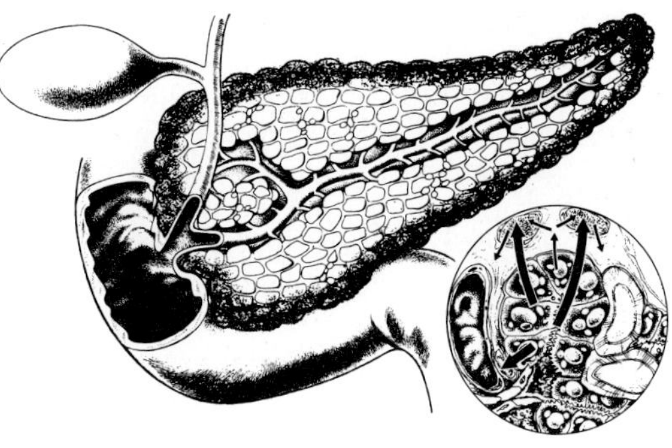

Fig. 32. Mantle fold pancreatitis, Kümmerle grade II.

Macroscopically, grade III of an acute lipolytic-proteolytic autodigestive pancreatitis as well as pancreatic apoplexy following bile reflux in common channel may be simulated. Histological detail in circle (see caption, Fig. 39): Partly compensated, partly decompensated edema; autodigestive lipolytic-proteolytic foci in adipositas interna in peripheral organ region. (ERCP is contraindicated; when performed, usually negative since, for technical reasons, the peripheral duct system is not visualized!)

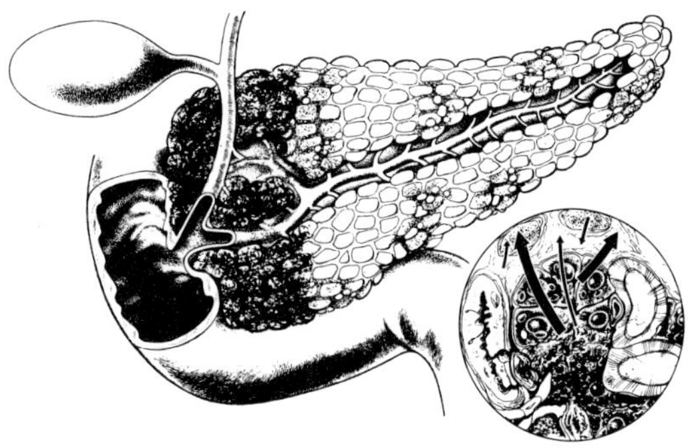

Fig. 33. Acute head pancreatitis, Kümmerle grade II.

Subtotal necrosis of head of pancreas and minimal lesions in regions of body and tail. Histological detail in circle (see caption, Fig. 40): Acinar necrosis, fat cell necrosis, marked topically circumscribed hemorrhages; decompensated edema in head region; compensated focal edema in body and tail regions. Minimal lesions may occur as forerunners.

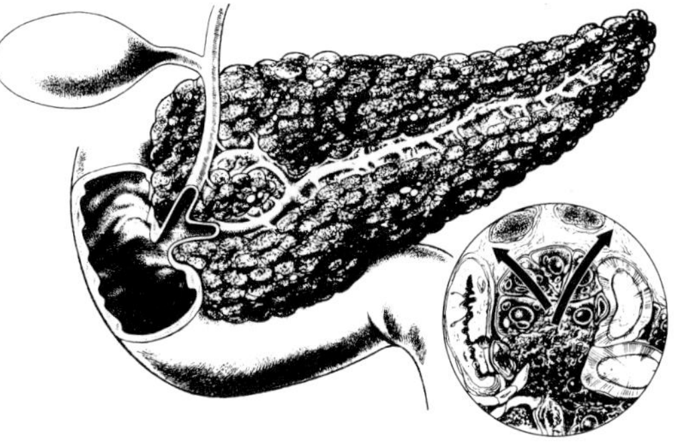

Fig. 34 = 31. In combination with concrement as shown in Fig. 12, pancreatic apoplexy as defined by Opie; Kümmerle grade III.

4.5.2   Dyschylia

This term was originally coined by Büchner [63] to denote disturbances of gastric juice secretion and was later applied to comparable diseases of the pancreas [40, 175, 427, 428]. With reference to the pancreas, it describes disturbances of the secretory process which may manifest themselves in the formation of secretions in the acinar cell itself, in the discharge of secretions, and in their transport through the ductal system [430]. If the term dyschylia is broadly interpreted, one may speak of a dyschylous juice edema with respect to the enzyme derangement [50]; even under physiological conditions this is macroscopically discernible at the peak of digestion and is histologically detectable as continual parapedesis into the interstitium [323], the extent to which this occurs is determined by the blood-juice barrier as well as the lymph-juice barrier. Its morphological substrate is the intimate contact between the lymphatic and capillary plexus and the excretory parenchyma in the periacinar region and that of the initial connecting ductules. Viewed against this background, the morphological components of the prephase of acute pancreatitis in conjunction with isthmic blockade take on special significance and underscore the morphogenetically close relations between chronic, chronic relapsing, and acute pancreatitis. Accordingly, it seems legitimate to propose, without sharp distinction from physiological parapedesis, a "morphological series" extending from minimal lesions to chronic and chronic relapsing pancreatitides and to disease forms marked by acute autodigestive exacerbations, distinguishing these from primarily biliary pancreatitis in a narrower sense. As in the case of the salivary glands, we may distinguish between an acinar and a canalicular dyschylia, or between a proteodyschylia and a hydrodyschylia [40, 430].

4.5.2.1   Proteodyschylia

This represents a disturbance of enzyme formation in the acinar epithelia; it results from damage to the intracellular protein metabolism: hypoproteinemia in the presence of an absolute nutritional deficiency, kwashiorkor or liver diseases; alcohol abuse (for details, see Chapter 3, Pathophysiology); hyperparathyroidism; model of "ethionine pancreatitis"; cytotoxic effects in electrolyte disorders, radiation damage, or virus infections.

These are the morphological substrates of acinar dyschylia:

hydropic vacuolar degeneration
loss of basal basophilia
acidophilic degeneration
necrosis of individual cells or groups of cells of acinar epithelium
dyschylous atrophy

(a) Hydropic vacuolar degeneration may be taken as a sign of acute oxygen deficiency of the cell [64]; its morphological substrate is composed of juxtanuclear vacuoles which dent the nuclear membrane. Resulting from hypoxia, hydropic vacuolar degeneration occurs at the inception of the proteolytic component of aLPP [473, 475] and initiates the "parenchymatous phase" of biliary pancreatitis [469]. Vacuolar and acidophilic degeneration are precursors of acinar epithelial necrosis.

   In the presence of hypoxia, the cells of the isthmic and connecting ductule epithelia undergo swelling with hydrops and loss of basal striation. The consequences are isthmic blockade and increased enzymatic parapedesis.

(b) Loss of basal basophilia follows the initial cellular swelling associated with zymogen extrusion and nuclear pyknosis; the cytoplasm undergoes a vesicular transformation due to vacuolation of the endoplasmic reticulum and depletion of ribosomes [101]. This finding is nearly always associated with acidophilic degeneration.

(c) The acidophilic degeneration is due to densification and separation of the protoplasm with destruction of ergastoplasm; loss of basal basophilia and acidophilic degeneration mark the transitional zone between autodigestive necrosis and intact acinar epithelia: the "target cell phenomenon." The changes culminate in the structural desintegration of all cell organelles; analogous changes are quite well known from the experimental model of "ethionine pancreatitis" or from general protein deficiency.

(d) Dyschylous atrophy encompasses a flattening of the acinar epithelia, changes in the nucleus-plasma relation, and dilation of the acini and connecting ductules. The acinar lumen contains thickened secreta (see Hydrodyschylia, 4.5.2.2); these alterations are the morphological equivalent of serious electrolyte disturbances and/or dehydration syndromes, as in uremia, ulcerative colitis, malabsorption syndrome, the dumping syndrome after a Billroth II gastric resection, mucoviscidosis, etc. [474].

Acinar cysts are considered indicative of the late stage of dyschylous atrophy.

4.5.2.2 Hydrodyschylia

The canalicular dyschylia in hypohydrochylia is associated with thickening of secretion and causes dilation of the acini and small pancreatic ducts with epithelial flattening. Thus, acinar dilation, thickening of juice, dissociation of the lobular structure, and pancreatic juice edema are typical of the early stages of metabolically induced pancreatitides. Local pancreatic alterations likewise lead to this form of dyschylia if the initial pancreatic ducts are displaced from their lymph channels and capillaries (widening of transmitter zone) owing to interstitial fibrosis associated with gastroduodenitis or as a late sequela of "associated pancreatitis." Thus, the dyschylia may be the consequence or the cause of juice edema and so occupies an intermediate position between the prephase and the trigger phase of acute pancreatitis. In its bland form, dyschylia is part of the precursory phase, involves minimal lesions, and is a forerunner of the juice edema [474]. Canalicular dyschylia compromises the necessary dilution of the secretion of a purely serous gland with a long excretory duct system or, as Becker [40] termed it, a "juice shower"; it is due to changes in water and electrolyte regulation, e.g., in uremia, burns, diarrhea, and the dumping syndrome following Billroth II gastric resection. In hypokalemia with increased loss of potassium from the cell and increased sodium and H_2O influx, the isthmic epithelial cells swell considerably, causing isthmic blockade and a consequent increase of parapedesis and juice edema. On the other hand, long-term secretory stimuli, as in alcohol abuse, lead to cell exhaustion with epithelial flattening and luminal dilation. Thickening of secretions, scaly dyschylia, and precipitation of microliths occur in the pancreatic ducts, e.g., in connection with proteodyschylia (see 4.5.2.1). This stage represents an intermediate station between chronic and acute pancreatitis in alcoholics. Owing to secretion against an obstacle (obstruction-hypersecretion theory of Dreiling et al., 1952, quoted by Wanke [476]) there is always a latent danger of juice edema and the possibility of acute exacerbation of the pancreatitis in the added presence of functional hypoxia of the acinar epithelial cells, notably in conjunction with adipositas interna (see discussion on components of prephase). This clinically very dangerous phase is generally preceded by a phase of hypersecretion and hyperhydrochylia (see Chapter 3); however this hypersecretion-"hyperchylia" is of no clinical significance [41]. Hypersecretion of the pancreas is seen in certain intoxications (e.g., sublimate poisoning) or after certain drugs (e.g., thiazides) and also in autonomically labile patients [35].

4.5.3   Edema: "Edematous pancreatitis"

At the beginning, edema may be a "reaction to overloading" when there is even physiologically an edematous tendency of the pancreas due to increased parapedesis, that is, release of secretions not into the ductal system but between the acinar epithelial cells via the acinus-shared basement membrane into the periacinar interstitial tissue.

A fact often overlooked in speaking of juice edema is that one has to distinguish between a juice edema of high danger and a vascular edema of generally little danger. In both cases, however, CT and sonography reveal a definite organ enlargement and the clinical picture may be one of "edematous pancreatitis;" the basic morphological processes are fundamentally different, however.

4.5.3.1   Acinar edema: Juice edema

Interstitial pancreatic juice edema, glassy edema, or Zoepffel's edema (Zoepffel, 1921) is one of the gravest morphological alterations in the early phase of every acute pancreatitis (BP, MP, LPP). Morphogenetically, this edema always results from dyschylia (see section 4.3, Biliary Pancreatitis). It is of importance in this connection that a periacinar interstitial system as a facultative space has direct contact with the terminal branches of the lymphatic system [18, 356, 358, 469]. There is also direct communication between the periacinar interstice and the portal circulation, a finding that is significant for the extent of associated damage to the liver parenchyma in the presence of enzyme derangement with or without lymph blockage (see Postphase). In the course of the development of acute pancreatitis the pariacinar interstices are considerably dilated; there is stasis in lymph and blood vessels. In later stages there is migration of erythrocytes into this interstitial system and into interstitial tissue generally (hemochylia) [402]. The enzyme derangement as a clinical-biochemical parameter of juice edema is brought about[101] by:

(1) expression of secretion via the walls of secretory tubules in the case of secretion against an obstacle;
(2) disseminated necrosis of individual cells (minimal lesions);
(3) parapedesis, i.e., escape of zymogen granules intercellularly, via the common acinar basement membrane, into the interstitial tissue.

Physiological secretion in response to stimulation is also characterized by increased parapedesis, hence a "tendency to edema formation" [131]. Thus, any abnormal strain on the secretory process can primarily result in an insidious organ transformation through a chronic, inveterate edema (see Prephase). We thus encounter edema both in the prephase and during the trigger phase of acute pancreatitis. The organ capsule is taut; there is conspicuous hyperemia! The macroscopic pattern resembles that seen at the peak of digestive secretory output. Because of the macroscopic appearance, the diagnosis "hemorrhagic pancreatitis" is undoubtedly made too often during surgery, particularly if only the external organ capsule and peri- or parapancreatic adipose tissue are taken into consideration.

As for the origin of the juice edema, it is often no longer possible to decide in the individual case whether the noxa striking the acinar cell arrives primarily from the periacinar and interacinar adipose-connective tissue (e.g., enzyme derangement starting by way of mast cell degranulation–shock model); in association with adipose tissue necrosis as autodigestive minimal lesions; as a continuation of neighboring processes, via the ductal and lymphatic systems–notably in the region of the pancreatic head–or hematogenously. Owing to the rapid chemically or autodigestively induced process of destruction during the morphogenesis of pancreatitis, these initial lesions are generally concealed at the time of examination, and mixed morphological findings predominate. Yet we know from experimentation [471, 476] and impressive autopsy reports that the pathogenetic pathways outlined above can in fact be differentiated, and that in the majority of cases a "group assignment" (BP, MP, LPP) is possible if account is taken of history and etiology, accessory and associated diseases, and the morphological substrate. It stands to reason that the percentage of idiopathic pancreatitides [88] cited in clinical surveys is relatively high, whereas it is rather low in pathoanatomical reviews [41].

It is essentially the drainage capacity of the intrapancreatic and extrapancreatic lymph system in conjunction with the local inhibitor potential which determines whether the "biochemical pancreatitis" with enzyme derangement in the broadest sense also becomes one in the morphological sense. The lymphatic passages function as a safety and overflow valve in the event secretory volume and pressure (see ERCP–watch for parenchymal phase!) become too high or the secretion has to overcome an obstacle.

4.5.3.2 Vascular edema

This form of edema, occurring in cardiac or portal congestion, changes progressively into an interstitial organ sclerosis. Increased afflux of blood (active hyperemia) with restricted blood efflux (e.g., combination with portal hypertension) leads to edema when lymph drainage is inadequate (e.g., in alcoholics with cirrhosis of the liver).

Toxic permeability defects in capillary and lymphatic vessels cause extravasation (capillary leak) with an added leuko-lymphocytic or predominantly hemorrhagic component; thus, the early stages of biliary pancreatitis (BP) are characterized by vascular edema [477]; the acute cytotoxic detergent effect of unconjugated bile acids results in coagulation necrosis of pancreatic duct epithelia and acinar epithelia affected by the reflux and in circulatory disorders of the ductular and periacinar vascular plexus. Subsequent stages are passed according to the reflux volume and the contamination period, and within a few minutes in fulminating cases; in the added presence of dyschylous-degenerative changes of the acinar epithelia, the enzyme content of the edema increases. The originally vascular edema turns into a mixed edema, the effect of which increasingly resembles that of juice edema (see discussion concerning late phase of BP); the chemical component of the organ destruction is then more and more overshadowed by the autodigestive lipolytic-proteolytic component.

The pathogenetic, hence also morphogenetic, difference between dyschylous and vascular edema is of critical importance, however, with respect to the causative noxa and, consequently, the prognosis and also with respect to the therapeutic approach (Figs. 35, 36, 37, 38, Plate IX).

Allergic-hyperergic diseases, increased protein decomposition in the presence of tumors or burns, and endogenous-exogenous intoxications likewise cause vascular edema. Added to this is the effect of vasoactive polypeptides, the two components not being exactly separable: burns with liberation of histamine, release of vasoactive polypeptides, shock, electrolyte shift, and protein decomposition with formation of so-called roast toxins.

The significance and effect of the kallikrein-kinin mechanism in acute pancreatitis and in postpancreatic shock are still variably evaluated [10, 80, 134, 178, 357, 358, 405] but local, short-term, and nonsystemic liberation of kinins [10, 80] presumably leads to a transitory vascular edema with a leukocytic component. The kallikrein-kinin system thus shares responsibility for an important component of pancreatitis–the substantial escape of fluid into the pancreas itself as well as retro- and intraperitoneally [347, 348, 412, 489, 490]. During the edematous phase of pancreatitis the lymph stream carries high concentrations of enzymes away from the pancreas and the peritoneal cavity [358, 490], an experimental observation which is now being translated worldwide into peritoneal dialysis, "peritoneal lavage" or directed drainage with irrigation (see pages 112, 121).

While kinins, apart from the aforementioned purely hemodynamic factors of vascular edema, play a critical role in the development of vascular edema, liberated mesenchymal and parenchymal lipolytic and proteolytic enzymes determine the autodigestive component of the edema [38, 407, 477].

In morphological terms, the edema represents the second phase of the morphogenesis of pancreatitis; it is preceded by the acinar dyschylia (see page 44). The dangers of further escalation are thus programmed beforehand, particularly if increased acinar necrosis is added to the purely degenerative dyschylous cellular changes. In spite of sonography and CT it is today hardly possible to estimate in clinical-biochemical terms whether this "edematous pancreatitis" will turn into an aLPP with or without hemorrhages, or whether in the head region it may be considered a bland variant of BP (see discussion concerning anatomical duct status, page 31). In the narrow sense, "edematous pancreatitis" corresponds to Kümmerle's severity grade I.

Pancreatic juice edema can end in aLPP, on one hand, and produce the late lipolytic-proteolytic phase of BP, on the other hand. Depending on the local inhibitor capacity and the drainage capacity of intra- and peripancreatic lymph channels and the number of prephase components that have already appeared, such as

(a) periductular and periacinar fibrosis,
(b) lymph blockage intramurally/cisterna chyli,
(c) pancreatic juice stasis,
(d) adipose tissue interposition
(e) vascular sclerosis,

the pancreatitis may remain "frozen" at the stage of *dyschylia* with *"minimal lesions,"* *edema* as "edematous pancreatitis," *circulatory dysfunction* with necrobiosis and autodigestion as relapsing chLPP; or in the case of massive, large-area *autodigestion* it may culminate in aLPP with or without hemorrhages.

4.5.4 Disturbed circulation

In addition to dyschylous alterations, secretion against an obstacle, and juice edema, a reduction in the rate of arterial blood flow, increased capillary permeability, and obstruction of venous reflux are regarded as factors potentially triggering an acute pancreatitis. Disturbances of pancreatic blood flow can have vascular, ductal (e.g., in BP or owing to chyme reflux), or acinar-cellular effects inasmuch as in shock or after maximal stimulation of secretion a functional hypoxia can lead to adipose tissue and acinar epithelial necrosis [384, 485, 491].

4.5.4.1 Functional circulatory disorders

4.5.4.1.1 Functional-neural
According to our present experimental and clinical-pathoanatomical knowledge, neural and neurovascular factors have only minor and additive effects, if any.

48

4.5.4.1.2   *Functional-hormonal-biochemical*

Hematogenously supplied vasoactive substances produce blood flow disturbances, to a dose-dependent degree, at the pancreatic periphery (e.g., epinephrine, norepinephrine). There are fluid transitions to digestive physiology in the blood flow-dependent pathophysiology of secretion. During digestion and a few minutes after administration of histamine, prostigmine, secretin, or pancreozymin the O_2 consumption and the blood flow rate of the pancreas become several times higher than in the state of rest. If this increase in arterial blood flow is no longer assured, e.g., in general ateriosclerosis, functional hypoxia and cellular necrosis result (see also discussions concerning dyspragia intermittens angiosclerotica, Orthner's disease; and age distribution of acute pancreatitis).

4.5.4.1.3   *Functional-physical*

Arterial hyperemia is associated with every acute inflammation; venous hyperemia, on the other hand, is observed in all states of congestion (cardiac defects, lung diseases with pulmonary hypertension, liver diseases with portal hypertension) (Table 12). Chronic congestion causes cyanotic induration of the pancreas with an increase of supporting and adipose tissue as well as atrophy of the excretory parenchyma. Leaving aside secondary circulatory disorders during the morphogenesis of acute pancreatitis as one of its phases, one finds interstitial pancreatic hemorrhages in portal vein congestion, after traumas, erosive hemorrhages of penetrating gastroduodenal ulcers, in connection with rupture of the lumbar aorta, and after death by suffocation.

4.5.4.1.4   *Shock hypoxia*

The significance of local acidosis for the provocation of acute autodigestive pancreatitis deserves special emphasis and has been adequately documented experimentally [42, 254, 469, 472]. Under physiological conditions, the optimal pH for the activation of trypsinogen to trypsin, as for the action of trypsin itself, is pH 7–9. Under pathophysiological conditions (acidosis, pH < 5), activation of trypsinogen to trypsin is likewise possible, as also through dissociation of the trypsin-inhibitor complex and subsequent autocatalytic activation of trypsinogen by trypsin (see Chapter 3). Very brief hypoxic phases thus become dangerous; a "spontaneous activation" of trypsinogen to trypsin and a chain reaction have to be expected [20]. Thus, aLPP is associated with autodigestive acinar epithelial necrosis around areas of initial fat cell necrosis (the "target cell phenomenon"), the origin of which can be traced to a decompensated acidosis [475]. Accordingly, a coincidence of prolonged shock and acute pancreatitis is seen more and more frequently [102, 152, 180, 384, 431, 474, 491]. Extensive operations generally entail increased cellular permeability, which is attributed to insufficiency of the microcirculation [49, 252, 321, 395]. The time of lipolysis, too, besides being determined by the enzyme level and the physical condition of the substrate, is pH-dependent [53]; thus, fat cells with hypoxic membrane damage are more vulnerable to the lipolytic enzymes. It is further worth noting in this connection that a massive degranulation of perivascular mast cells takes place in shock and during the trigger phase of acute experimental pancreatitis, and this within a few minutes after administration of the noxa [145, 477]. The human shock organs are characterized by a particularly high metabolism during activity and performance, hence a high oxygen consumption. In shock, the liver, kidneys, pancreas, stomach, duodenum, and lungs play a vital role; because of the possibilities of intensive therapy, the lung is clinically becoming the "limiting factor," while complications involving the other organs are becoming increasingly controllable by therapy. These organs have high enzyme contents. There is the group of lysosomal enzymes in liver and kidneys, and the ones bound to zymogens in the pancreas; a third group to be mentioned is the mast cell content of the organ. Next to the human subcutis, the lung, stomach and duodenum, and the pancreas have the highest mast cell content per cubic millimeter [235, 433, 470]. As a human shock organ, the pancreas is not only one of the enzyme-rich organs but also has a high mast cell content. Besides histamine and heparin (also serotonin in rats), the mast cell granules contain trypsin, chymotrypsins, phospholipase A and active lipids (fatty acids, unsaturated lipids [66, 92, 242, 433]). The mast cell granules have a great deal in common with the lysosomes of other cells [8] and play an important role in intracellular and extracellular protein digestion. This interpretation explains findings made in lower animals (e.g., individual fish species [383]), in which atypical mast cells of the gastrointestinal tract are more like the acinar epithelial cells of the pancreas than the mast cells of higher species. During the phase of edema and disturbed circulation in acute pancreatitis, therefore, the enzyme potential of the tissue mast cells of the pancreas, as well as the liberation and activation of acinar enzymes, is of considerable importance.

A comparison of the pancreatic changes occurring in metabolic pancreatitis [254, 471] and in hemorrhagic shock reveals fundamental differences in their time course [101, 102, 411]:

(a) Metabolic noxae damage the cell organelles involved in protein synthesis primarily and the mitochondria secondarily.

(b) Vasuclar-hypoxic noxae as a rule cause structural disruption of the mitochondria initially and produce damage to the other cell organelles secondarily.

Whereas complete hypoxia causes secretory performance to cease, partial ischemia induces a discharge of zymogen granules, intensified basophilia of the ergastoplasm, vacuolar degeneration, nuclear edema, and necrosis of individual cells—the changes observed in acinar dyschylia [250, 431].

4.5.4.2 Vascular-organic circulatory disorders

4.5.4.2.1 Arteriosclerosis

Arteriosclerosis of the pancreatic vessels causes marked fibrosis of the organ and reduction of the excretory parenchyma in conjunction with adipose tissue proliferation, on one hand, while on the other hand the manifestation of acute autodigestive pancreatitis is significantly related to it [476] (see also discussions on age distribution of acute pancreatitis, arteriosclerosis as a component of the prephase, low incidence of acute pancreatitis in children, and the aged-over-50 risk factor [372]). There are close interrelations with uremia, in which sclerosis of interlobular pancreatic arteries and interstitial edematous fibrosis occur in addition to canalicular and acinar dyschylia. Sclerosis of pancreatic vessels is considered significant in that it adds to the factors that combine to produce functional insufficiency; in other words, with increasing age short-term local hypoxia is more likely to provoke autodigestive minimal lesions. This finding is in agreement with the clinical observation that the risk of a life-threatening form of pancreatitis rises abruptly after age 50 [372].

4.5.4.2.2 Arteritis

Arteritis is a rarity, in contrast to the high incidence of degenerative changes in pancreatic vessels, and is only of anecdotal interest in connection with acute pancreatitis [476].

4.5.4.2.3 Allergic-hyperergic

Whereas an abundance of data can be cited as evidence of a positive correlation between degenerative vascular changes and acute autodigestive pancreatitis, we have to rely on hypotheses about a presumed allergic-hyperergic pathogenesis [476]. The multitude of experimental studies on these questions may be divided into three groups [100]:

(1) Induction of a serum, histamine-peptone shock, resulting in the pattern of "edematous pancreatitis";
(2) Induction of an Arthus reaction (general sensitization and subsequent injection of antigen into pancreatic duct or vein; a "hemorrhagic-necrotic pancreatitis" results);
(3) Induction of a Shwartzman phenomenon, also resulting in a "hemorrhagic-necrotizing pancreatitis".

To apply these experimental data to the human situation, however, is highly questionable from the point of view of general pathology. There are critical morphogenetic differences between a local Shwartzman phenomenon, for example, at the site of the pancreas and acute autodigestive pancreatitis: In Shwartzman pancreatitis the small- and medium-caliber vessels in the vicinity of the pancreatic ducts are the sites of the initial lesion – it thus bears a morphological resemblance to biliary pancreatitis – whereas autodigestive lipolytic-proteolytic pancreatitis affects the acinar epithelia themselves, and this in a perifocal pattern around areas of adipose tissue necrosis. Also, the hemorrhages in Shwartzman pancreatitis are due to primary vascular lesions (see also discussion concerning the type of biliary pancreatitis, 4.3), whereas they result from proteolytic and elastolytic rhexis in autodigestive pancreatitis; furthermore, the at times considerable thrombus formation must be considered a primary event in the former but a secondary one in the latter. "Toxins" demonstrable in the serum in "allergically-hyperergically" induced pancreatitides are vasoactive polypeptides (see Chapter 3, Pathophysiology); the titer of these "noxae" generally corresponds to the severity of the pancreatitis; edema, ascites and hypotension are attributed to these polypeptides. Experimental findings by Seelig and Seelig [426], according to which cytolytic complement is responsible for the initial damage to the acinar cell membrane in acute pancreatitis, require confirmation and verification before their relevance to the morphogenesis of pancreatitis can be assessed.

4.5.5 Necrobiosis, necrosis (autodigestion)

Necrobiosis is intravital death of nucleated cells and groups of cells under pathological conditions. The nuclear atrophy develops only after a certain lapse of time. The end result is a complete breakdown of all structures, called necrolysis. Karyolysis and karyorrhexis are indicative of increased proteolytic activity and are pH-dependent. In nuclear atrophy and chromatolysis the protein component of the nucleoprotein is split off by proteases, while polynucleidases eliminate the nucleins themselves.

The common morpholigical substrate of chronic and acute autodigestive lipolytic-proteolytic pancreatitis (ch/aLPP) is the phenomenon of acinar and ductular dyschylia. This dyschylia is induced metabolically or by hypoxia; it causes damage to the cell organelles involved in protein metabolism or to the oxidative apparatus of the acinar cell. Differences in the magnitude of the damage extend as far as group necrosis. Besides clearing reactions with interstitial inflammation, insidious organ transformation and fibrosis, lipolytic-proteolytic autodigestive foci develop as minimal lesions. Their number depends on the scope of the preceding interstitial adipose tissue proliferation; patterns of "chronic pancreatitis" thus develop which as a *prephase* lay the morphological basis for aLPP in as many as 85% of cases; by the same token, the histological components of acinar dyschylia appear in a parenchymally "exaggerated" form in acute pancreatitis.

The *sites* of the *trigger phases* of acute autodigestive pancreatitis with necrotized acinar epithelial cells near areas of fat cell necrosis are shown semischematically in Fig. 39, Plate X and Fig. 40, Plate XI:

Fig. 39, *early phase,*

Fig. 40, *late phase.*

The acute exacerbation is triggered:

(1) *hematogenously* via direct damage to the acinar epithelia, the action being directed at the organelles of the constructive and functional metabolism (metabolic form), or at those of cell respiration (hypoxic form) in shock and hypoxia;

(2) *lymphogenously* from topically contiguous organs;

(3) *mesenchymally* through release of mast cell enzymes, by an indirect hematogenous route as a septic-metastatic excretory inflammation with the vascular-connective tissue apparatus as the action site, i.e., mesenchymally, in contrast to hematogenously, where the parenchyma itself is the action site;

(4) *canalicularly* due to bile or chyme reflux and through bacterial or parasitic ascension.

Up to a certain stage of the organ transformation and parenchyma-destroying atrophy, the danger of acute exacerbation is morphologically inherent in every chronic pancreatitis. On the other hand, there is a direct relation between the zymogen content of the pancreas and the severity of the pancreatitis [486, 487, 488]; a burnt-out pancreas devoid of enzymes is no longer capable of pancreatitis.

4.5.5.1 Enzymatic necrosis

The phasic course of acute pancreatitides is demonstrable chiefly in the autodigestive ch/aLPP forms, the nearly specific morphological substrate being determined by the organ's own enzymes.

4.5.5.1.1 *Lipolytic enzymes*

Necrosis of adipose tissue critically determines the pattern of the pancreatitis. The pancreatic lipase as the "key enzyme" of the autodigestion received notable attention even around the turn of the century [476]; much of this knowledge fell into oblivion since then. In the '60s and '70s experimental studies revived, confirmed, and supplemented old findings. It could be shown that the pancreatic lipase decisively stamps the morphological picture of chLPP, actuates the "trigger mechanism" of subacute exacerbation, and also contributes greatly to the effects of biliary or chyme reflux.

4.5.5.1.2 *Lipase*

This enzyme acts on the phase interphace of the oil-in-water emulsion, which has a high H^+ ion concentration [53]. According to electron microscopic studies [358, 471], this "phase boundary surface" is obtained at the cell membrane if general acidosis (see discussion concerning shock) with an increased H^+ ion concentration brings about a loosening of the cell membrane structures; the lipase is then able to attack its lipid components; subsequently, intracellularly stored fat becomes the substrate of lipolysis. The triglyceride cleavage and liberation of fatty acids produces local acidosis and ensuing activation of proteolytic proenzymes, notably trypsinogen, and subsequent activation of prephospholipases by active trypsin. This chain reaction explains the morphological phenomenon of the exact perifocal localization of autodigestion around areas of fat cell necrosis (minimal lesions, lipolytic-proteolytic autodigestive foci, target cell phenomenon). There also is a direct correlation between the extent and number of areas of adipose tissue necrosis and intra- and peripancreatic adipose tissue interposition or apposition (see Prephase, Table 9a). Fat necrosis results from soap formation, complexes being formed by calcium ions and free fatty acids that are liberated from triglycerides under the catalytic action of lipase; these are often discernible as "calcium splashes" with the naked eye and thus frequently provide a diagnostic "guide rail" during operations. Activation of lipase does not occur; it is already present in the cell in active form; construed teleologically, its substrate is lacking in the acinar cell under physiological conditions. This is not true for phospholipase A or the proteases, which are accordingly stored as zymogens or proenzymes. However, the timing of lipolysis depends on the pH, the enzyme level (significance of adaptive lipase increase, e.g., model of "cortisone pancreatitis" [485]) and on the physical condition of the substrate (finely or coarsely emulsified, hence relations to BP). The rate of hydrolysis is promoted by bile salts and Ca^{++} ions [130]. Bile as a detergent increases the surface area of the substrate and so enlarges the action site of the lipase (= "enhancement of effect"). Unconjugated bile acids, moreover, have a cytotoxic effect, destroy the cell membrane, and thus make intracellular substrate accessible to the lipase in adipositas interna: positive interrelations between overweight (adipositas interna), cholelithiasis, and ch/aLPP (Table 6). The role of lipase in the morphogenesis of lipolytic-proteolytic pancreatitis is described in Table 14.

Table 14. Significance of pancreatic lipase for development of nonbiliary pancreatitis (lipolytic-proteolytic pancreatitis [LPP]).

1. Apparent positive correlation exists between obesity and severity of LPP
2. Inter- and perilobular fat cells become the initial substrate of active lipase and focus of LPP
3. Necrotized acinar epithelial cells are found at first in the immediate vicinity of necrotized fat cells ("target cell phenomenon")
4. Intraductular instillation of lipase causes acute pancreatitis of the LPP type only in obese animals
5. Experimental, spontaneous, and iatrogenic "cortisone pancreatitides" are of the LPP type
6. Apparent positive correlation exists among adrenal function, obesity, and pancreatic enzyme activity
7. Bilaterally adrenalectomized rats do not develop LPP following intraductular administration of fat emulsion as a lipase substrate
8. Hormonally active adrenocortical tumors can be associated with LPP

4.5.5.1.3 *Phospholipase A (with subgroups [80])*

This enzyme is present as a zymogen [20, 94, 120]; even minimal amounts of active trypsin are able to convert prephospholipase A to the active enzyme. It is a hydrolytic enzyme which splits off a fatty acid from the phospholipid; lecithin becomes lysolecithin. As with lipase, Ca^{++} ions and bile salts increase the rate of hydrolysis. The cytotoxic effect of the phospholipase A reaction products, lysolecithin and lysocephalin, is due to their incorporation into the cell membrane [93]. When a combination of phospholipase A and an 0.4% sodium taurocholate solution, which by itself exhibits no appreciable cytotoxic activity [487, 488], is experimentally injected into the pancreatic duct system, it produces hemorrhages over small areas and perivascular parenchymal necrosis within 60 minutes [151, 408]. Intraductular administration of lysolecithin as a 2% solution [83, 408] causes parenchymal necrosis-coagulation necrosis after some time. However, account has to be taken of the morphological development [487]: A few minutes after the lysolecithin installation an excessive juice edema sets in and the acinar epithelial cells prove to devoid of zymogens (!) even while no necrosis is discernible at first; however, the uninitiated may mistake chromatin-dense nuclei for necrosis. A conspicuous general hyperemia then leads, within 2 hours, via prestasis and peristasis with erythrocyte sludging, to extensive thromboses of the intrapancreatic and, in part, peripancreatic vascular plexus. Subsequently, karyorrhexis and karyolysis set in by way of hypoxia-induced dyschylia. The morphogenetic course shows that in terms of the organ destruction the effect of phospholipase is a "secondary effect."

The human bile is rich in lecithin; lysolecithin is formed rapidly in conjunction with phospholipase A. Unconjugated bile acids and lysolecithin attack the membrane so that their effects on the pancreatic duct and acinar epithelia become additive after bile or chyme reflux. In the presence of bile acids (see discussion of problems with head pancreatitis in presence of accessory pancreatic ducts, Section 4.2) phospholipase A also causes mast cell degranulation [307] (dysoria of the histamine type); a similar effect can be produced by a combination of kallikrein and phospholipase A [13]. The combined effects of lipolytic enzymes, bile, and mast cell enzymes demonstrate once again that the "pure form" of biliary pancreatitis as understood by Opie and Halstedt, with impacted papillary stone, reflux, and common channel, is the exception and that mixed forms dominate the morphological picture of reflux pancreatitis.

As pointed out above (see Section 4.5.4.1.4) the pancreas occupies a zwitter position in shock; we have to distinguish between postpancreatitic shock with the systemic sequelae of enzyme derangement = the disease of pancreatitis (see Complications, Table 25) and the fact that the pancreas must be considered one of the shock organs. Among the toxic substances released during the disease of pancreatitis, phospholipase A as well as lipase plays an important role systemically. In particular, the lecithin component of the pulmonary surfactant becomes a substrate; the hydrolysis of the surfactant lipids of the lung alveoli and of lipids in the capillaries [343] accounts for the high incidence of pulmonary insufficiency and shock lung in acute pancreatitis [491].

4.5.5.1.4 *Proteolytic enzymes*
The proteolytic enzymes trypsin, chymotrypsin, elastases, cathepsins and carboxypeptidases are of pathophysiological importance in the context of autodigestion.

4.5.5.1.5 *Trypsin, chymotrypsins*
In terms of the pathomorphological performance of proteolytic enzymes during the trigger phase of acute pancreatitis it is noteworthy that active trypsin is not only unstable as such [130, 131] in a neutral environment, i.e., during the stage of pancreatic juice edema ("edematous pancreatitis"), but is at this point optimally inactivated by the specific trypsin inhibitor (Forell et al., 1965). In this phase, therefore, further chain reactions can still be prevented. Acinar epithelial cells with a balanced energy metabolism are fortified against autodigestion [42]. An essential precondition is restriction of cell respiration with protein denaturation. The primary development in evolving pancreatitis of the LPP type accordingly is fat cell necrosis with general hypoxia, resulting in local acidosis following triglyceride cleavage, hypoxic vacuolation of perifocal acinar epithelia, and in the stages of dyschylia up to autodigestive necrosis of parenchymal cells (Figs. 41–44, Plate XII). Minimal lesions, too, probably remain localized as a rule by protease inhibitors that are initially present in the pancreas in high concen-

trations (specific trypsin inhibitor, α_1-antitrypsin, α_2-macroglobulin [28, 31]). We encounter the familiar biological phenomenon of a quantitative reaction (see discussion of balance or imbalance between defensive and aggressive factors, Pages 18, 40). Only when the intraorganic inhibitor capacity [21] is exhausted can the chain reaction, viz., acute exacerbation, e.g., after minimal lesions, no longer be arrested. In other cases, such as the biliary variant, the very first biochemical-physical phase is associated with collapse of micro- and macrocirculation [469] so that the inhibitor potential is "overrun" from the outset and can no longer prevent the autodigestive postphase or late phase.

Minute amounts of active trypsin are capable of autocatalytically transforming trypsinogen into trypsin. Independently of activators, the increased parapedesis and local acidosis around areas of fat cell necrosis, or general systemic acidosis, as in shock or diabetic coma, can provoke the spontaneous activation of trypsinogen.

Experimental studies have yielded largely identical findings regarding the morphological effects of trypsin and chymotrypsin; they are dose–dependent. Low concentrations cause juice edema, hemorrhages, and parenchymal necrosis [38, 83, 468, 488]. The juice edema develops in a few minutes. Hemorrhages, thromboses, and vascular erosions follow later. The hemorrhagic component is attributed chiefly to an effect of elastase [101, 146], other autors ascribe it to the effect of kinins [449]. Inasmuch as trypsin catalyzes the activation of the other enzymes that become effective in autodigestion, except lipase, the parenchymal necrobiosis and the degradation of collagenous and elastic fibers as well as the associated vascular component are essentially initiated through trypsin.

The acute autodigestive pancreatitis is thus triggered via:

(1) *lipase* – triglyceride cleavage – local acidosis – trypsinogen cleavage – enzymatic chain reaction = aLPP type;

(2) *acidosis* – activation of trypsinogen – chain reaction (e.g., autodigestive late phase of BP).

Most investigators are in agreement about the morphological effect of trypsin (experimentally verified) up to the development of a more or less hemorrhagic juice edema. In more recent studies greater importance has been attached to the protease-antiprotease imbalance [28, 137]. Even in the edema phase, hemorrhages, in some cases extending over large areas, have the added mechanical effect of structural disruption, so that a critical hypoxic component supervenes. In keeping with this development, the acinar epithelia in the vaicinity of the pathways of the edema are vcuolated; the initially focal enzyme derangement quickly spreads to adjoining lobules (enzymatic "flying sparks"). Over areas of fresh autodigestive necrosis, the proteolytic digestive component can be demonstrated histotopochemically in frozen sections [47, 48] by the Todd method of "fibrinolysis autographs" [453] (Fig. 45, Plate XII). During the rapidly progressing destructive process, karyolysis with appearance of "perforated nuclei" proves characteristic of the proteolytic component [477].

As may be expected, intrapancreatic interstitial juice edema as well as lymphogenous, hematogenous, and transcapsular enzyme derangement with associated cavitary effusions (ascites, pleural, percardial effusions) yields high levels of active proteolytic enzymes [490] and vasoactive polypeptides [28, 31]. On the basis of this experience, peritoneal dialysis ("peritoneal lavage") and directed drainage and irrigation find increasing use as essential therapeutic measures in acute pancreatitis.

4.5.5.1.6 *Elastase*

This enzyme is decisive for the vascular component of autodigestive pancreatitis [101,

146, 322], including destruction of elastic and collagenous fibers, vascular erosion with extensive hemorrhages, and thrombosis. As after administration of trypsin or chymo-trypsin, autodigestive parenchymal necrosis develops besides. The various mesen-chymal and parenchymal alterations are due to the elastolytic as well as the proteolytic component of this enzyme.

4.5.5.1.7   Carboxypeptidase A and B

These enzymes supplement the protein breakdown initiated by trypsin, chymotrypsins and elastase. Morphological characteristics shared by the proteolytic enzymes are the phenomenon of dysoria* (see Table 15), a barrier disorder (impairment of blood-pan-creatic juice and lymph-pancreatic juice barriers), and the consequent development of edema which, with the added capillary leakage, always culminates at the peak of the pancreatitis in a mixed edema having dyschylous and vascular components.

The lypolytic and proteolytic enzymes involved in the autodigestion have their own specific morphological substrates (Table 15).

Table 15. Enzyme – Substrate – effects

Enzyme	Substrate	Effect (see Chapter 3)
Lipase	Triglycerides	Fat cell necrosis
	Intracellular	Local acidosis after triglyceride
	Intraductular	cleavage, intra-acinar lypolysis
		Loosening of cell membranes
Phospholipase A_1, A_2	Cell membrane phosphatides	Lysophosphatide formation,
Trypsin	Lecithin of bile	membrane destruction, dysoria
	Activation of:	Coagulation necrosis
	Trypsinogen	Dysoria
	Chymotrypsinogen	
	Proelastase	
	Prekallikrein	
	Prephospholipases	
	Procarboxypeptidases;	
	Denatured scleroproteins	
Chymotrypsins	Denatured scleroproteins	Coagulation necrosis
		Dysoria
Carboxypeptidases	Denatured scleroproteins	Coagulation necrosis
		Dysoria
Elastase		
a) Elastolytic component	Elastic, collagenous fibers	Elastocollagenolysis
b) Proteolytic component	Denatured scleroproteins	Coagulation necrosis
		Dysoria
Kallikrein	Kininogens	Kinin liberation, Dysoria

4.6   Appendix: Infectious pancreatitis

Infectious pancreatitides proper do not fit into the context of the above data on biliary (BP) and autodigestive lipolytic-proteolytic (LPP) pancreatitis. Pizzecco [362] calls the

---

* Dysoria, from the Greek horos = limit.

inflammatory disease forms "pancreatitis" in the strict sense of the word and uses the term "pancreatosis" for the autodigestive manifestations. From the morphological viewpoint such a distinction is questionable since the BP and LPP types described are also inflammatory in nature, if only secondarily.

Primarily infectious pancreatitis manifests itself chiefly in the vascular-connective tissue system and therefore is of a mesenchymal character, viz., serous, seropurulent, purulent-abscess-forming during the acute stage, and lymphocytic-plasmacytic with added activation of the mesenchymal cell component in more chronic disease forms (see Chapter 2).

4.6.1 Bacterial

As an "associated pancreatitis" [100] it occurs during and after infections and is looked upon as a metastatic or excretory pancreatitis or evaluated as an infectious-allergic process [173, 427]. Morphologically, one finds equivalents of chronic interstitial lymphocyte-plasmacyte infiltrations with more or less pronounced interlobular or perilobular as well as periductular fibrosis, without any evidence of added components of autodigestion. In cases in which abscesses or the picture of pancreatitis phlegmonosa have been described [173], late complications of primary LPP or BP generally are involved.

Bacterial toxins hardly play a primary role in the development of parenchymal necrosis [191, 464, 476]. However, chemical-biliary as well as autodigestive parenchymal necrosis is quickly followed by a bacterial superinfection from adjoining organs (see Chapter 8), as a result of which late complications with abscess and fistula formation may arise.

In exceptional cases, septic excretory metastases in the pancreas have been seen after staphylococcal, streptococcal, and coli infections and after typhoid and paratyphoid fever or amebic dysentery, occasionally involving the excretory and incretory parenchyma in "heterodigestion" [471].

4.6.2 Viral

The finding of chronic parenchyma-destroying interstitial pancreatitis following virus infections has been made in comparative pathology [469]. The source of infection may be coxsackieviruses or the mumps virus; in human pathology such cases have been described almost exclusively in children [161, 429]; they are of interest only as case reports and clinical history. The coxsackie and the Newcastle viruses and the viruses responsible for epidemic hepatitis are considered particularly pancreatotropic (Fikry, 1968; Acir, 1968). The morphological substrate for coxsackievirus is similar to that in "metabolic ethionine pancreatitis" [471]; the organelles of anabolism and functional metabolism, hence the protein synthesis of the acinar epithelial cells, is affected. The consequence is acinar dyschylia (see Section 4.5.2.1) and associated inflammatory interstitial clearing reactions.

Summary
This attempt at a systematized presentation of the pathogenesis and morphogenesis of acute pancreatitides is based on experimental data and on analysis of a multitude of individual pathoanatomical observations in patients who died of acute pancreatitis. It is a reflection of the clinical diversity of the pancreatitic disease and provides feedback for diagnosis and therapy.

Chapter 5 – Clinical Features of Acute Pancreatitis

Two large groups of entirely different pathoanatomical disease processes and disease forms are subsumed under the clinical term acute pancreatitis: *acute edematous* and acute *hemorrhagic-necrotizing pancreatitis* with all their variants and possible overlaps.

Acute pancreatitis is a threat particularly for heavy eaters and drinkers ("gourmand pancreatitis").

In its severe form the disease begins suddenly, violently, and dramatically without warning signs. In about one-third of the cases it sets in after a sumptuous meal, rich, fat foods, and ingestion of alcoholic, often chilled beverages with a sudden severe pain that immediately reaches a peak and occasionally causes loss of consciousness. This "annihilating pain" in the upper abdomen is usually accompanied by severe vomiting and marked agitation.

There is an immediate or very rapid transition to status pancreaticus. This is characterized by intensity of subjective symptoms, early onset of changes in the general condition and, particularly, signs of shock with few clinical findings.

Milder variants present comparable but, on the whole, substantially less severe symptoms.

5.1 Subjective symptomatology

5.1.1 Pain as cardinal symptom in acute abdomen: The special case of acute pancreatitis

General prefatory note to elucidate the symptom of pain:
The most important biochemical and pathoanatomical pain-provoking mechanisms are:
1. Distention of muscular hollow organs (stomach, intestine, gallbladder, kidneys/urinary tract).
2. Metabolic disorders, notably metabolic acidosis.

From this we can draw the most important diagnostic inferences regarding varying sensations of pain (type and quality of pain in relation to time and changes) (Tables 16, 17, 18; Figs. 46, 47, 48).

In muscular hollow organs increased muscle tone with hypermotility provokes pain. The types of pain originating from visceral organs are called visceral. They pass via viscerosensory nerve fibers in the autonomic nervous system to the spinal ganglia and hence to the posterior horn cells of the spinal cord. Pain sensations in the serosa-lined abdominal cavity (peritoneum), on the other hand, travel along different pathways. Painful impulses emanating from the parietal peritoneum are not conducted through fibers in the autonomic nervous system but via the somatosensory fibers of the spinal nerves. Pains from the peritoneum are therefore experienced or described as somatic. Somatic pain is constant and becomes increasingly sharp and, because of the peritoneal irritation from the disease of the organ, is precisely localized or felt by the patient at the site of its provocation. This means that the pain is visceral in character so long as the diseased organ alone is affected. Localization of the pain thus makes possible an approximate diagnosis of the organ. If the initially localized organ disease spreads, however, and diffusely extends to the peritoneum, the pain assumes a somatic character. The simultaneous changeover to the motor ganglion leads to irritation and consequent reflex guarding. The persistent, continuous irritation brings about a constant contraction of the abdominal wall musculature, as e.g., in the rigid abdomen of patients with perforating ulcer and diffuse peritonitis.

A rapidly spreading peritonitic irritation always entails, because of the underlying septic peritonitis, changes in general condition, and especially circulatory changes with signs of shock. In a colic or mechanical ileus, therefore, the disease picture in its initial stage (!) – with as yet no peritonitis (migration peritonitis) – is characterized less by circulatory chances than by pain-induced restlessness and posture.

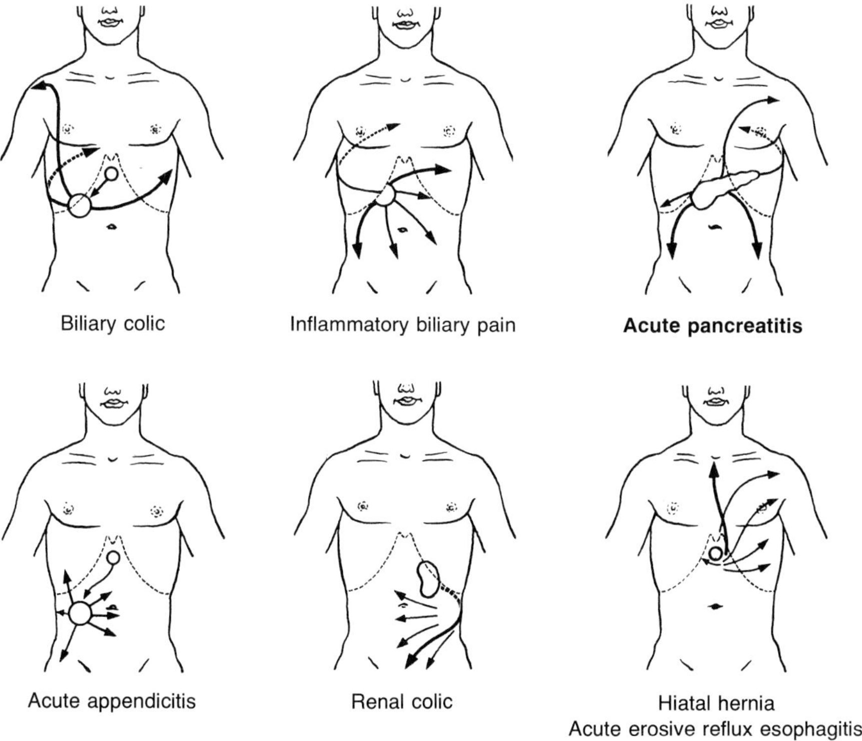

Fig. 46. Topography of pain in different abdominal diseases.

Table 16. Analysis of different pain qualities in acute abdomen

1. Colics	Violent, undulating pain involving the autonomic nervous system, e.g., vomiting
2. Somatic pain	Stabbing, boring, persistent pain; localizable upon irritation of peritoneum, e.g., by palpation or tapping
3. Visceral pain	Dull, deep, intermittent pain, difficult to localize; irritation of autonomic nervous system
4. Phrenic pain	Irritation of branches of phrenic nerve and consequent radiation to shoulder region (shoulder pain, e.g., in cholecystitis)

Table 17. Organmorphology and Topography of pain-provoking organs

Pain originating from
1. the parenchymatous organs
2. the muscular hollow organs of the digestive tract
3. the genitourinary organs
4. the peritoneum.

Topography of pan in acute abdomen: *Pain regions* according to *incidence*
1. Epigastrium
2. Mesogastrium – umbilical region
3. Right hypogastrium
4. Right lower abdomen
5. Left lower abdomen
6. Left hypogastrium
7. Suprapubic area

The indicative symptom of pain has to be viewed in relation to the general condition, and the crucial diagnostic and therapeutic conclusions must be drawn:
1. Every progressive intraabdominal inflammation manifests itself by the transformation and displacement/migration of pain (Table 16).
2. The isolated occlusion of a single hollow organ causes intensified activity with colicky pain but relatively little deterioration of the general condition. These systemic reactions are therefore absent in all simulated peritonitic processes.

Note: A chance from visceral to somatic pain is an important diagnostic and developmental criterion.

Examples
penetrating/perforating ulcer,
gallbladder colic with or without subsequent cholecystitis (hydrops, empyema),
gallbladder perforation.

Cholecystitis initially entails painful inflammatory reactions and spastic contractions with or without colic that are experienced as visceral pain. Not until the inflammation has spread beyond the organ boundaries does the so-called somatic pain (parietal pain) develop (Table 18, Figs. 47, 48).

Table 18.   Diseases simulating peritonitis, without actual peritonitic irritation (pseudoperitonitis)

I

Pleura– Mediastinum	Diaphragmatic pleurisy, angina pectoris, myocardial infarction, acute pericarditis, pulmonary infarction, spontaneous pneumothorax, blunt chest trauma
Pancreas	Chronic, locally uncomplicated pancreatitis
Kidneys– Urinary tract	Inflammations, colic due to calculi, cyst, nephroptosis
Urinary bladder	Cystitis, retention ("full bladder")
Vessels	Abdominal angina, mesenteric infarction, mesenteric thrombosis, aneurysms, rupture, hemorrhage, intestinal wall hematoma or retroperitoneal hematoma in anticoagulant therapy, rupture of spleen or liver
Abdominal wall	Muscle lacerations, hematomas, trauma (contusions)
Genital	Myoma, ablatio placentae; torsion of ovarian cyst, testis, genital tumor

II

Metabolic disorders	Diabetic precoma (pseudoperitonitis diabetica), uremic coma, hypokalemic coma, hypocalcemia, tetany (differential diagnosis pancreatitis!)
Intestinal spasm	Intoxications (lead or thallium); porphyria!
Severe vomiting	Acute glaucoma, tabes dorsalis, meningitis, migraine, herpes zoster, Meniere's disease, labyrinthitis, sunstroke, hyper- or hypoparathyroidism, Addison's disease, pregnancy, psychogenic vomiting, Acute liver congestion, addisonian crisis, collagen diseases
Systemic diseases (heart, lung, circulation)	Pneumonia, Pleurisy, angina pectoris, abdominal angina
Intestinal inflammations	Typhoid, dysentery, mesenteric lymphadenitis, tuberculosis, pseudotuberculosis (Pasteurella infection), Echinococcus
Specific general infections	Gastric crises in tabes

Whereas the isolated inflammation of an organ in the abdomen makes itself felt by a transformation, intensification and displacement of the pain with general reactions and, in particular, systemic effects, the occlusion of a hollow organ alone (biliary, renal colic, mechanical ileus) is initially characterized only by an isolated, highly painful colicky sensation. Beyond the process in the organ, blood loss or septic intoxications due to peritonitis or neglected ileus give rise to life-threatening, often irreversible general injuries which are associated with a high mortality rate despite intensive medical treatment of these secondary sequelae (paralytic ileus, respiratory and renal failure) and successful surgery of the organ.

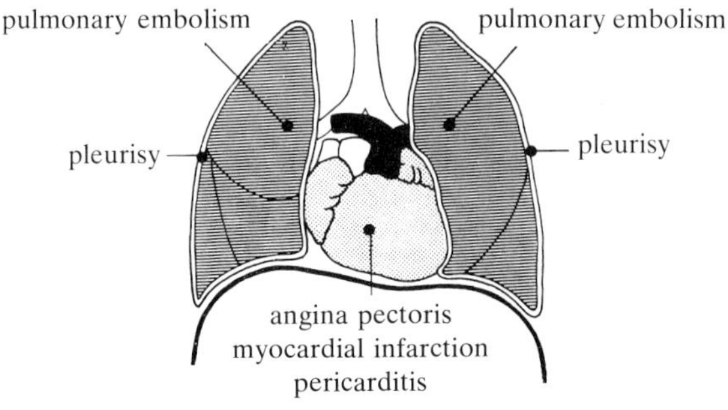

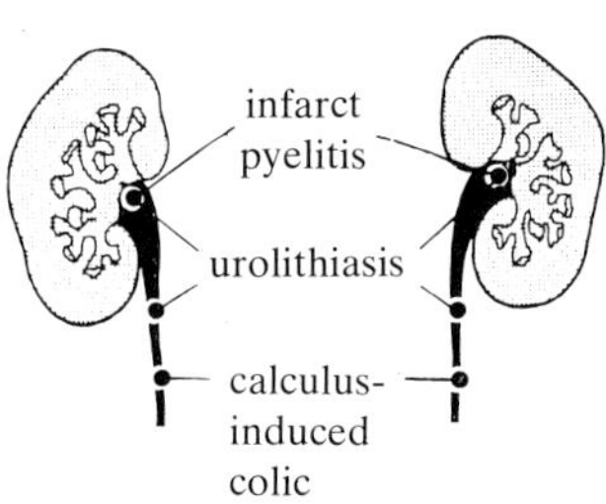

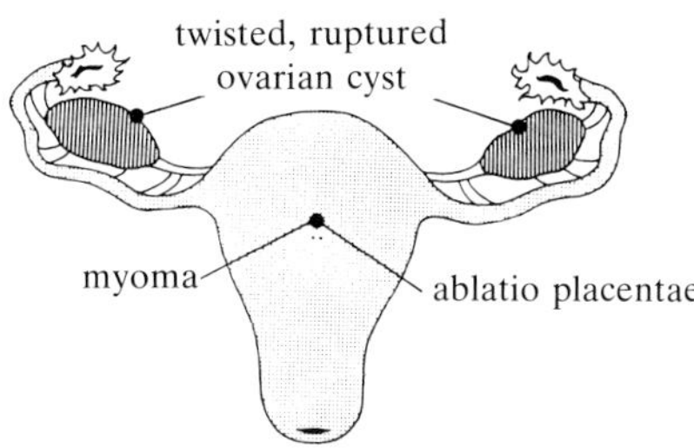

Fig. 47. Extraintestinal and retroperitoneal organ diseases with signs of peritoneal irritation = peritonism (pseudoperitonitis).

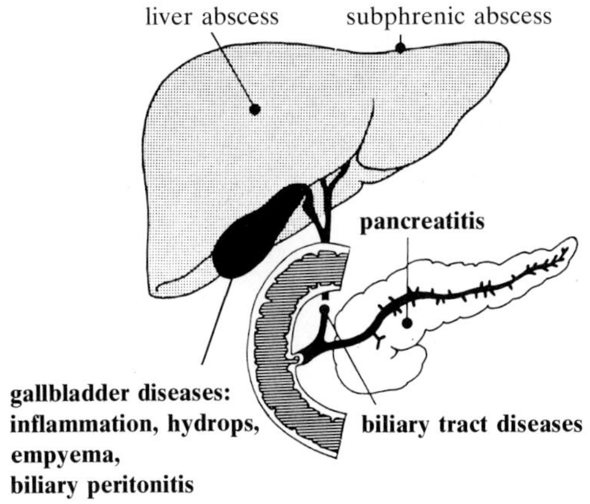

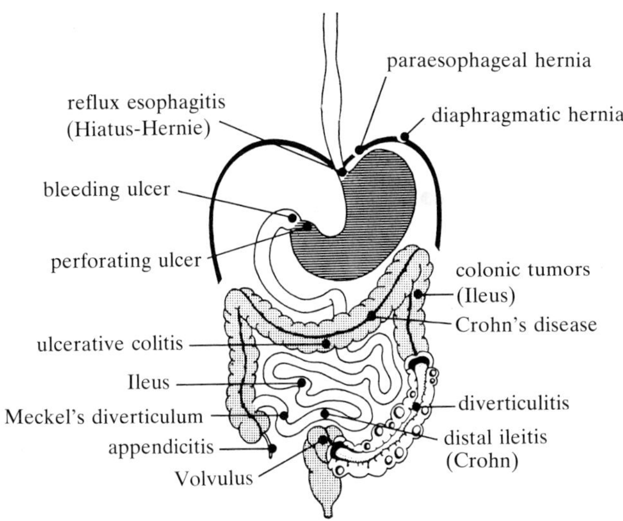

Fig. 48 a. Acute abdomen. Differential diagnosis – topographic organ diagnosis of acute abdominal diseases with genuine peritoneal irritation and pain.

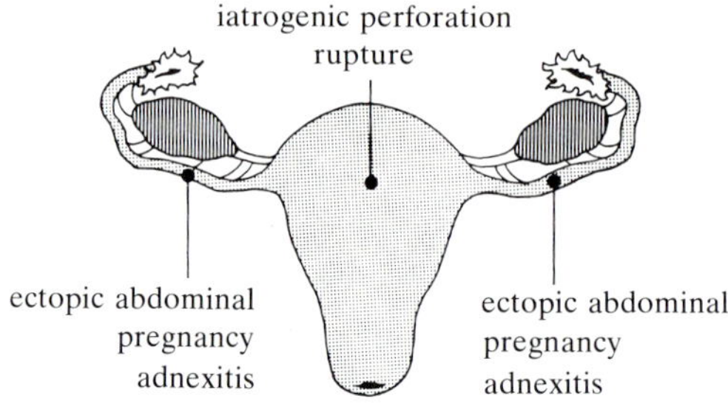

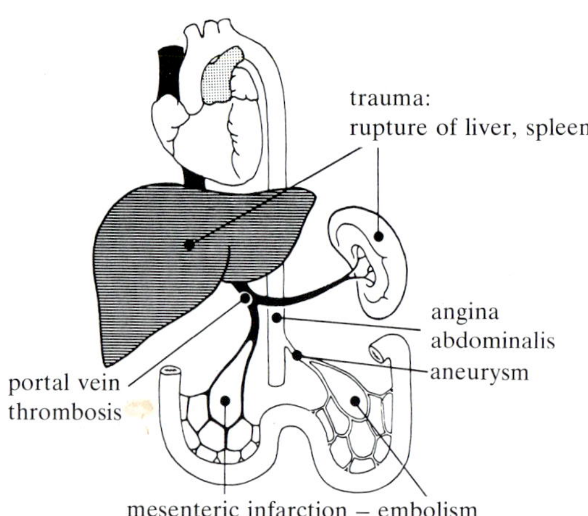

Fig. 48 b. Acute abdomen. Differential diagnosis – topographic organ diagnosis of acute abdominal diseases with genuine peritoneal pain.

All the special and combined general effects described above are present in complex fashion in pancreatitis. With its specific autodigestive inflammatory process, it is thus one of the diagnostically and therapeutically most difficult and problem-causing gastroenterological diseases.

The pain is caused by an edematous distention of the pancreatic capsule and by massive release of kinins and increase of permeability. The patient screams and moans with pain and cannot find enough superlatives, such as "dagger-like" and "agony," to describe it; the face is distorted with pain, a facies almost typical of pancreatitis.

Furthermore, this pain produces a state of anxiety in the patient. In 70% of the cases the pain is localized in the upper abdomen, the medial epigastrium. It radiates in various directions, generally toward the rear, dorsally or deep inside, from the epigastrium to the back.

In some cases the pain is greater on the right than on the left. A left-sided pain which radiates dorsally and to the left is suggestive of a disease of the tail of the pancreas, whereas radiation to the right shoulder is more indicative of disease of the pancreatic head with possible involvement of the gallbladder and the bile ducts and radiation to the right diaphragm (irritation of phrenic nerve on the right).

Epigastric pains suggest involvement of the pancreatic isthmus and corpus.

Not infrequently the patient complains of a persistent pain of remarkable intensity which does not respond to analgesics. This pain causes a typical antalgic posture to be assumed, the so-called "pancreas position" or hunched-up "praying" position. This contrasts with anginal attacks in which the patient assumes a rigid, half-seated position. By the "praying or crouching position" he tries to obtain relief from the pain by bending forward and by hunching up – the knee against the chin and the fists pressing into the upper abdomen.

5.1.2   Vomiting

Eighty percent of patients with acute pancreatitis have to vomit. This is primarily a reflex action. Large quantities of gastric contents – first food remnants, then bile, and finally mucus and pure gastric juice – are discharged. Rarely, the vomitus has a feculent odor and in exceptional cases it is bloody as a sign of hemorrhagic gastritis. However, vomiting brings no relief to the patient but aggravates his anxiety.

5.1.3   Subileus

A functional subileus with retention of feces and flatus is often present, and is initially confined to the upper jejunum and transverse colon.

5.1.4   Dyspnea/polypnea

Dyspnea and polypnea are observed particularly in anxious patients with jerky respiration. Dyspnea as such is not characteristic of acute pancreatitis. It occurs with all upper abdominal pains that restrict diaphragmatic motion.

5.2 General symptomatology

This is equally significant for evaluating the severity of the pancreatitis. The patient's state of anxiety is particularly noticeable. Marked agitation, cyanotic discoloration of the face, cold extremities, and perspiration-drenched facies point to severe worsening of the general condition and circulation. A certain mental confusion is sometimes apparent. This initial state of agitation can turn into a real mental aberration with attacks of delirium due to an enzymatic encephalopathy, as shown by patches of cytosteatonecrosis detectable in the brain and meninges. The possibility of a withdrawal delirium has to be taken into account in the differential diagnosis.

5.2.1 Parameters of shock

The intensity of the shock depends on the severity of the acute pancreatitis and on the time at which the patient is examined. Moderately pronounced symptoms of shock are seen in 50% of all patients, and severe shock in 15% of cases of acute pancreatitis. Especially noticeable is the extreme variability of pulse and blood pressure (note shock index/shock disposition!).

Frequently, the following course is taken:

The arterial blood pressure rises immediately after onset of the "attack." The pulse rate remains the same; occasionally it is slightly elevated. Both the systolic and the diastolic pressures are increased by 10–40 mm Hg above normal levels. The increase may last 2–3 hours and is then characteristic of the severity of acute pancreatitis and not infrequently associated with a flush syndrome. For the differential diagnosis, however, it is very seldom indicative.

Soon thereafter a tachycardia sets in, while at the same time the arterial blood pressure decreases. In such cases the pulse rate is about 120–150/min. The discrepancy between the pulse and the arterial blood pressure is one of the most important presumptive signs of the severity of pancreatitis (shock index!). If all the symptoms of the disease fail to diminish after the institution of therapy, and the pulse rate remains above 100, this means that the pancreatitis is spreading.

5.2.2 Body temperature

The body temperature is normal at the beginning and then rises slightly, rarely above 38.5° C. The dissociation between apyrexia and leukocytosis with polymorphonuclear leukocytes is of diagnostic value, particularly if it occurs within the first 6 hours.

5.2.3 Subicterus

A subicterus of the sclera develops in the first 48 hours in about 30% of all cases of acute pancreatitis, or is already present during that period. The cause of this subicterus varies. It may be due to obstruction of the distal common bile duct by edema of the pancreatic head (distal choledochal stenosis), or a choledochal calculus may be impacted in the ampulla of Vater, or a toxic hepatitis may be present.

5.3   Clinical symptomatology

5.3.1   Abdomen: Inspection

Inspection of the abdomen shows that this is distended but abdominal respiration is still good. Although only the epigastrium or the right or left upper abdomen is distended initially, a diffuse, more or less painful, pasty muscular defense slowly spreads out.

5.3.2   Abdomen: Cutaneous signs

The "acute abdomen" in acute pancreatitis is accompanied by various cutaneous signs (cutaneous phenomena). However, they appear in only about 10% of cases, on the 3rd or 4th day, taking various forms.

5.3.2.1   Cyanotic spots

These lend a marbled appearance (Halsted's sign) to the abdominal wall.

5.3.2.2   Blue coloration of umbilical region: Cullen's sign

Bluish spots in umbilical region.

5.3.2.3   Turner's sign

Bluish or yellowish ecchymotic spots are sometimes seen in the umbilical region and in the flanks. They are characteristic of the development, spread, and retroperitoneal resorption of a hematoma (Turner's sign). This sign is not specific, however, since it can appear also upon rupture in extrauterine pregnancy or, exceptionally, in the course of a hemorrhagic small bowel gangrene.

5.3.2.4   Rubeosis

This reddish skin discoloration, notably in the area of the pancreatic head (i.e., in the right upper to medial abdomen), is observed in about 25% of the cases. It is due to the vasodilating effect produced in the initial stage by the kallikrein-kinin system (see Chapters 3 and 4).

5.3.2.5   Warren's sign

Warren has pointed out that the blue discoloration of the umbilicus often is the result of an edematous infiltration, the early appearance of which is suggestive of considerable pancreatic damage and prognostically unfavorable.

5.3.2.6   Patches of cytosteatonecrosis

Spots of cytosteatonecrosis on the thorax and in the pleura as well as on the buttocks have also been reported.

5.3.3   Abdomen: Palpation

Palpation of the abdomen causes pain. On the whole, the abdomen presents a pasty, pliable resistance. Only in 30–40% of acute pancreatitis cases is there moderate guarding, which is localized exclusively in the upper abdomen. There is no characteristic muscular defense (as in perforating duodenal ulcer, for example). Milder forms are characterized by a weak muscular defense and cessation of intestinal peristalsis as evidence of subileus or transient intestinal atony. More pronounced guarding and persistent ileus are associated with the severe forms. Also to be mentioned is the left-sided subcostal pain observed by Mallet-Guy, and the pain in the left posterior costovertebral angle between the tail of the pancreas and the vertebral column. This location of the pain is considered pathognomonic by Mayo-Robson.

5.3.4   Abdomen: Percussion

Percussion of the abdomen reveals a distinct meteorism but the hepatic dullness remains. The Goblet-Guyot sign, which is characterized by a sound strip running across the upper abdomen, stems from an isolated dilation of the transverse colon.

5.3.5   Ascites and abdominal exudation

Ascites and abdominal exudation (note differential diagnosis!) are often present to varying degrees and account for the dullness demonstrable by percussion in the lower and lateral abdomen. These changes develop early. Biochemical analysis of ascitic fluid and exudate (protein and enzyme contents) is most important for differential diagnosis. Diagnostic peritoneal lavage discloses high amylase and lipase concentrations similar to those found in the pancreatogenous pleural effusions described below (see Chapter 3).

Table 19. Acute pancreatitis: Incidence of clinical symptoms

	%
Severe abdominal pain	90–100
Nausea, vomiting	70– 90
Meteorism	70– 80
Subileus	60– 80
Ascites	50– 70
Elevated temperature	40– 50
Shock	30– 50
Subicterus	30– 50
Muscular defense	30– 40
Respiratory insufficiency	20– 30
Pleural effusion	15– 20
Shock kidneys	10– 20
Clouded sensorium–pancreatic encephalopathy	10– 15

5.3.6 Abdomen: Auscultation

The incidence of the most important clinical symptoms is shown in Table 19.

Auscultation of the abdomen reveals that the characteristic intestinal sounds are absent, reflecting disturbed intestinal activity.

5.3.7 Thorax: Percussion

As a general rule, percussion of the thorax should always be performed as well in order to detect or rule out a pleural effusion in time. Pleural effusions, usually but not always on the left side, are found in approximately 20% of all severe cases of pancreatitis. Occasionally, there is pleural effusion only on the right side; in a few cases it occurs bilaterally. Puncture yields a serofibrinous, often slightly blood-tinged fluid with increased amylase and lipase values in sharp contrast to at times normal blood values (see Chapter 6).

A pericardial effusion is also seen in exceptional cases.

5.3.8 Special case: Posttraumatic pancreatitis

Clinical features and diagnosis: The symptoms are variable and singularly dependent on the extent of other intraabdominal and extraabdominal injuries. In patients with multiple injuries, diagnosis is therefore extremely difficult in pancreatic trauma or a possible posttraumatic pancreatitis. Early symptoms, as in every acute pancreatitis, are slight guarding confined to the upper abdomen and deep tenderness on palpation, with the pain occasionally radiating between the two shoulder blades. Analysis of the pain by palpation and subjective description is hampered by the pain due to abdominal contusion. Review of the history as well as the early interval with few symptoms that has been described by many authors is important. Just as in nontraumatic pancreatitis, there is nausea and vomiting in connection with absent intestinal peristalsis due to functional ileus. However, as in nontraumatic pancreatitis, the course may also be fulminating, contrasting with the early stage presenting few symptoms.

Timely and accurate interpretation of the disease picture is possible only by continuous observation. Frequently, however, hidden pancreatic lesions or a posttraumatic pancreatitis are not uncovered until an exploratory laparotomy or autopsy is performed.

Posttraumatic pancreatitis is particularly serious after trauma in the region of the pancreatic head; postraumatic pancreatitis in the body or tail of the pancreas is prognostically more favorable because of the greater ease of operation. In these cases, too, the clinical signs are not pertinent or reliable for evaluation of the anatomical status of the organ.

Chapter 6 – General and Special Diagnosis

Besides examinations prooving diagnosis many supplementary measures are necessary in order to evaluate the disease course and the prognosis and to arrive at therapeutic conclusions, especially regarding the prevention and treatment of complications (see also Chapter 10.2, Table 30). Most important for the diagnosis is the detection of increased serum levels of lipase and/or amylase together with corresponding sonographic changes and clinical findings (Table 20).

Table 20. Laboratory investigations for demonstration of acute pancreatitis and for evaluation of course and prognosis and for detection of complications

Demonstration of disease	Evaluation of course and prognosis, detection of complications
	Scheme of Ranson et al. [373] (cf. Chapt. 8, Table 24) Diagnostic peritoneal lavage Methemalbumin
Serum lipase	
	(persistent enzyme derangement) ⟶ (e.g. in pseudocysts)
Serum and urine amylase (pancreatic isoamylase)	
Phospholipase A ⟶ (increase proportional to severity of disease?)	
Trypsin – RIA (enzyme specific for pancreas but determination unsuited for primary diagnosis because of the time required)	Creatinine and BUN in serum Total protein and albumin in serum CBC (particularly Hb, Hct, WBC, platelets) Coagulation tests Blood sugar Lipids Electrolytes, especially Ca^{++} Bilirubin, transaminases, LDH, alkaline phosphatase, γ-GT
	pO_2, pCO_2, acid-base metabolism

6.1   Laboratory investigations

6.1.1   Tests for demonstration of acute pancreatitis and their diagnostic value

The enzymes synthesized by the pancreas are also found in the serum under physiological conditions, if in low concentrations. In acute pancreatitis they pass into the blood directly or indirectly, via the lymphatic system or after absorption from exudates, and become detectable in the blood in high concentrations. Even in acute pancreatitis, however, the biological detection of active proteolytic enzymes in the serum is possible only in exceptional cases since they are inactivated by protease inhibitors. They are therefore detectable only by radioimmunoassay (e.g., trypsin). This technique, because of the time required, is not suitable for the routine diagnosis of acute pancreatitis. Most commonly, amylase and lipase concentrations are determined in the serum and exudates, and amylase is determined in the urine. Attention has been called recently to the importance of phospholipase A determination, especially with respect to the course and prognosis [420].

6.1.1.1   Amylase and lipase

Even though the reliability of lipase or amylase determination is affected in some measure by the assay method employed, serum lipase seems to be a more sensitive, pancreas-specific parameter than α-amylase [292]. Lipase determination is generally also somewhat more demanding than amylase determination [see 238, 381].

As a rule, one finds serum lipase and amylase levels several times greater than normal values in acute pancreatitis. There is no relation between the magnitude of the increase in the concentrations of these enzymes and the severity of the disease. False positive as well as false negative results may be obtained. Thus, amylase and lipase concentrations may be increased in renal insufficiency (due to reduced renal excretion of the enzymes), biliary tract diseases (associated with pancreas disease?), perforating ulcer, or ileus (increased absorption of enzymes from small intestine?), for example. Increased secretory pressure in the pancreatic duct system due to increased tone of the spincter of Oddi (e.g., upon opiate administration [224]) or strong stimulation of the pancreatic secretion rate (see discussion of evocative tests [354]) can likewise produce increases in serum enzyme levels without pancreatic disease being present or resulting.

In addition, elevated amylase levels are found in acute parotitis (even without associated pancreatitis), for which reason some authors recommend determination of the pancreatic isoamylase. The presence of *macroamylasemia,* too, has to be considered at increased serum amylase concentrations. While the amylase molecules are normally eliminated via the kidneys, the formation of molecular complexes of amylase molecules, glycoproteins or polysaccharides in macroamylasemia produces a molecular size that either precludes or restricts renal filtration, with the result that the serum activity of the enzyme increases. This finding by itself is of no pathognomonic value. However, there has been a report about a patient with "symptomatic" macroamylasemia in idiopathic sprue [187]. In this case the amylase molecules formed complexes with IgA, which disappeared on a gluten-free diet. To rule out macroamylasemia as the cause of an increase in serum amylase, urinary amylase (which is not increased in macroamylasemia) or serum lipase should be determined. The repeatedly advocated determination of amylase clearance in relation to creatinine clearance [495] does not appear to provide any additional diagnostic information on this point or for the diagnosis of pancreatitis in general [82].

A small increase in serum lipase concentrations reportedly occurs during heparin therapy by way of activation of lipoprotein lipase, the activity of which can at times be codetermined in a lipase assay [155]. In contrast to urinary amylase, urinary lipase cannot be measured reliably.

Normal serum levels of amylase or lipase do not definitely rule out acute pancreatitis, particularly if much of the organ has been destroyed by the disease, or there is an acute episode of an advanced chronic pancreatitis, or if the diagnosis is not made until several days after the onset of the disease. Determination of the enzymes in pleural exudate, in ascitic fluid, or in the lavage fluid is therefore especially important for identification and prognosis of the disease (see Chapter 3).

6.1.1.2   Other enzyme determinations

The radioimmunoassay of *serum trypsin* affords the advantage of pancreatic specificity. However, elevated levels are found, as for amylase and lipase, also in renal insufficiency [264] and may be expected as well in associated reactions of the pancreas or increased enzyme absorption (e.g., in ileus). The long time elapsing between blood collection and availability of the test result (36 hours) makes this assay method appear unsuitable for routine use. The same applies to radioimmunoassays of *α-chymotrypsin, elastase* and *carboxypeptidase B* [224].

In view of the pathophysiological significance of phospholipase A in acute pancreatitis [343], the determination of *serum phospholipase* A_2 is recommended [420]. Inasmuch as significantly higher phospholipase A_2 concentrations were found in patients with hemorrhagic-necrotizing pancreatitis than in patients with a less severe form of pancreatitis, this assay might in the future play a key role in both diagnosis and prognosis (course, complications). Yet studies on a larger scale seem necessary for a definitive evaluation of this method.

6.1.2   Studies for evaluation of course and prognosis and for detection of complications

6.1.2.1   Course and prognosis

Despite numerous attempts it has not been possible so far to arrive at a reliable assessment of disease course at the start of the illness by establishing specific criteria. The *scheme of Ranson et al.* [373] is considered helpful (Chapter 8, especially Table 24). This uses the patient's age and 10 laboratory parameters at the beginning of treatment or 48 hours after the diagnosis. A severe disease course is assumed if more than three prognostically unfavorable signs are found. Mortality is believed to increase in proportion to the number of these parameters. They include *hypocalcemia,* which is taken to be prognostic per se (see 6.1.2.2).

McMahon et al. [311] recommend *diagnostic peritoneal lavage* (see Chapter 7), in which the demonstration of "ascites" (more than 10 ml or dark brown discoloration) and the extent of hemorrhagic discoloration of the lavage fluid serve as immediately available parameters for course and prognosis. By this method a severe course was correctly predicted in 72 % of cases, and a mild one in 95 %, whereas on the basis of clinical evaluation a severe course was correctly predicted at that time in only 39 % of cases. After 48 hours, a severe course was correctly predicted in this study in 82% of cases by use of the Ranson scheme, in 83% by clinical evaluation, in 56% by the presence of hypocalcemia (<2.1 mmol/liter), and in 29% by determination of methemalbumin; a mild course was correctly predicted in 79% (Ranson), 100% (clinically), 83% (hypocalcemia), and 88% (methemalbumin determination). Diagnostic peritoneal lavage is not suitable for detecting late complications (pseudocysts or abscesses), however [310].

Schröder et al. [420], who credit determination of *phospholipase A₂* with prognostic significance (significantly higher values in patients with hemorrhagic-necrotizing pancreatitis; see 6.1.1.2), found increased methemalbumin levels in only two of five patients with confirmed hemorrhagic-necrotizing pancreatitis. By contrast, Lankisch et al. [273], on the basis of observations in 62 patients with acute pancreatitis, regard *methemalbumin determination* as a prognostically valuable, if not pancreatitis-specific parameter for differentiating the hemorrhagic-necrotizing form and the edematous form of the disease and in regard to the onset of complications. Differences in methodology and/or with respect to the timing of the assay presumably account for these divergent assessments of methemalbumin determination (see also Geokas and Rinderknecht [148]).

6.1.2.2 Detection of complications

Besides intensive clinical monitoring of the patient, the clinical chemistry parameters need to be closely followed if complications are to be detected early (see Chapter 10, specifically Table 30).

Special attention has to be paid to disturbances in fluid and electrolyte metabolism; the fluid balance, circulatory status, particularly CVP (central-venous-pressure), serum electrolytes and renal function should be continuously monitored. Hypokalemia besides hypovolemia may develop as a result of edema, ascites, retroperitoneal fluid and electrolyte loss, and ileus. The common complication of acute renal failure (see Chapter 8), on the other hand, leads to hyperkalemia.

Hypocalcemia can be due to adipose tissue necrosis with intracellular calcium deposits and to a shift in extracellular and intracellular Ca^{++} concentrations, decrease of protein-bound Ca^{++}, increased release of calcitonin (hyperglucagonemia), and to increased enzymatic degradation of the parathyroid hormone (see Chapter 3.4).

One should watch for hypophosphatemia, which has also been reported in acute pancreatitis (see Chapter 3; Jacobsen et al. [232]).

Hypercalcemia suggests hyperparathyroidism, hence the precipitating cause of such a case of pancreatitis.

Measurements of hemoglobin and hematocrit provide clues to intraabdominal blood loss or gastrointestinal bleeding (e.g., in erosive gastroduodenitis or in bleeding from varices of the gastric fundus resulting from segmental portal hypertension due to splenic vein thrombosis). On the other hand, a rise in hematocrit, in conjunction with other parameters (e.g., decrease of CVP), may reflect a volume deficiency.

According to Ranson et al. [373], a leukocytosis of more than 16,000 pro µl is prognostically unfavorable (see above and Chapter 8, specifically Table 24). A decrease of serum protein, notably albumin, can be caused especially by ascites or pleural exudation (see Chapter 3).

Disturbances of carbohydrate metabolism (see Chapter 3) can lead to hyperglycemia and glucosuria. Determination of bilirubin, alkaline phosphatase, γ-GT, transaminases, and LDH is necessary to investigate the etiology of the disease but also with a view to side effects and complications (e.g., choledochal stenosis due to edema of head of pancreas).

Acute renal failure due to shock or enzymatic parenchymal necrosis manifests itself in a decrease of urine excretion with increases of serum creatinine and BUN (blood urea nitrogen). Note should also be taken of pathological urine findings (proteinuria, erythrocyturia, leukocyturia, casts).

Pleuropulmonary complications (shock lung, pleural effusion) manifest themselves in clinical chemistry by a drop in pO_2 and pCO_2. Besides determining arterial pO_2 and pCO_2, shifts in the acid-base metabolism should be watched (also in view of possible metabolic acidosis). Blood coagulation defects (hypocoagulopathies, thromboses, embolism, disseminated intravascular coagulation) are uncovered by checking the coagulation status (platelets, thrombin time, fibrinogen, Godal test antithrombin III).

Last but not least, the serum lipids should be monitored since patients with familial hyperlipoproteinemia have a higher incidence of acute pancreatitis. Moreover, increased lipolysis in acute pancreatitis brings about a rise in the serum lipid concentrations. Finally, chronic alcohol consumption can provoke pancreatitis as well as secondary hyperlipoproteinemia. The disease course will have to be followed in order to arrive at the correct diagnosis [291].

In conclusion, we are referring once more to the summary of laboratory investigations in Tables 20 and 30.

6.2   Diagnostic ultrasonography

Sonography of the upper abdomen can be quickly performed, is safe and presents no hardship for the patient, and is therefore well suited for monitoring the course of acute pancreatitis. The method is highly accurate [109, 261, 444, 500]. It can shed light on etiological factors and on the severity and course of the disease, and can also detect complications and associated diseases (e.g., fatty liver) (Table 21). Cholecystocholedocholithiasis is the most important causative factor in acute pancreatitis. Cholecystolithiasis is detectable by sonography in nearly all cases (91–99%), as is a congestion in the bile duct system (92–97% [425]). The detection of choledochal concrements, however, often fails–particularly with smaller concrements–for technical reasons (retroduodenal course of common bile duct often overlaid with gas). The same is true for the detection of small tumors closely related to the head of the pancreas (e.g., papillary carcinoma). In finding the cause of a bile duct obstruction, therefore, sonography is only between 50% and 80% accurate (see Schwerk [425] for review).

Obesity (limited depth of penetration of sound waves) and a heavy accumulation of gas in the intestine (total reflection of sound waves) can hamper examination of the pancreas or even render it impossible. Thus, visualization of a morphologically unremarkable pancreas, for example, succeeds–despite preparation of the patient–in only about 80% of cases [444]. In acute pancreatitis, the sensitivity of sonography, as of computed tomography (CT), amounts to 80% [261]. It should be borne in mind, however, that the informative value of sonography is codetermined in large measure by the experience of the examiner (Table 22).

Table 21. Value of diagnostic ultrasonography in acute pancreatitis

Indication	Findings to be expected	Evaluation
Clues to etiological factors	Cholecystolithiasis	91–99% accuracy [425]
	Bile duct congestion	92–97% accuracy
	Causes of obstruction (e.g., choledocholithiasis)	50–80% accuracy
	Tumors relative to head of pancreas (periampullar tumors)	small tumors can be overlooked
Evaluation of severity and course	Pancreatic edema Partial pancreatic necrosis Total pancreatic necrosis	sensitivity about 80% [339] (monitoring disease course!)
Detection of complications	Abscesses, effusions (pleural, pericardial), pseudocysts, ascites, pathways of necrosis, fistulas, shock kidneys, splenomegaly	follow-up studies needed for detection!
Aid in choosing endoscopic papillotomy or surgical intervention	Choledocholithiasis with congestion of bile ducts and reflux pancreatitis; progression of disease despite exhaustive conservative therapy; pseudocysts with compression or displacement of adjacent organs; abscesses	See Neher et al. [339]

Fig. 49 shows a normal sonographic record of the pancreas. Pancreatic edema is characterized by enlargement of the organ and decrease of sonic reflexes (Fig. 50). Unsharply demarcated low-echo to echo-free areas are noted in necrosis (Fig. 51 a). Spread of necrosis beyond the pancreas (e.g., to renal region) is sonographically detectable (Fig. 51 b, "Necrotic pathways") (see also Chapter 8). Pseudocysts are also echo-free but sharply demarcated from their environment (Figs. 52, 53).

Table 22. Diagnostic value of sonography and computed tomography (Lackner et al. [261])

	Sonography	Computed tomography
Advantages	1. Variable scanning direction 2. Differentiation of solid and liquid structures 3. Determination of dynamic parameters (e.g., vascular pulsation) 4. Bedside examination 5. Hazard-free examination 6. No radiation 7. Low cost of examination These advantages allow disease course to be closely followed	1. Comprehensive anatomic-topographic overview 2. Measurement of tissue densities 3. Functional diagnosis after iv administration of contrast medium (e.g., detection of necrosis) 4. Broad applicability (not confined to organs) 5. Standardized recording technique (quality independent of examiner) 6. Image contents more easily understandable by inexperienced physicians 7. No interference from skeletal or intestinal gas overlay
Disadvantages	1. Image interference from large differences in impedance (e.g., air/parenchyma, bone/parenchyma) 2. Limited depth of penetration of sonic beam (e.g., in obesity) 3. Examination difficult after recent surgery 4. Image quality dependent on experience of examiner	1. Kinetic artifacts with uncooperative patients 2. Poor organ demarcation in very slim patients 3. Radiation load 4. Costly examination Because of these disadvantages the examination cannot be repeated to often

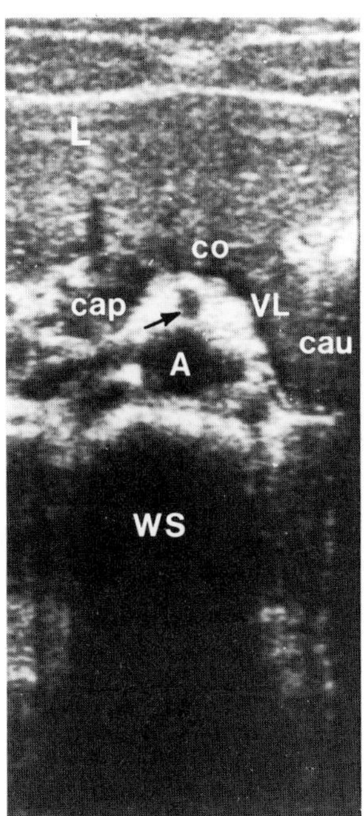

Fig. 49. Normal sonographic record of pancreas. A = aorta; → = superior mesenteric artery; cap = head of pancreas; co = body; cau = tail; L = liver; VL = splenic vein; WS = vertebral column.

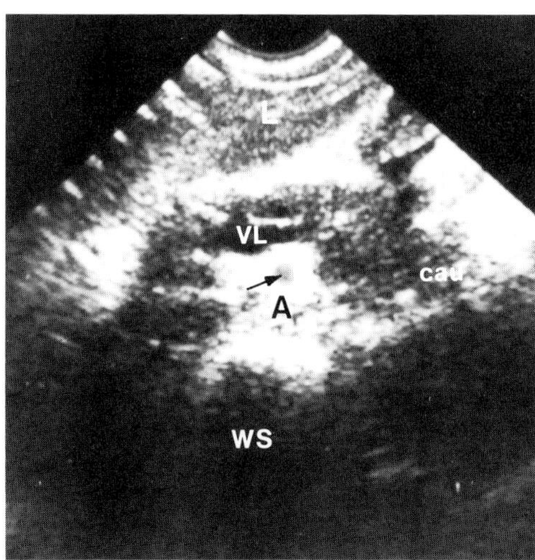

Fig. 50. Edematous pancreatitis. A = aorta; → = superior mesenteric artery; cau = tail of pancreas; L = liver; VL = splenic vein; WS = vertebral column. Supplied by courtesy of A. Gebauer, M.D., Radiological Clinic, University of Munich (Director: Prof. J. Lissner, M.D.).

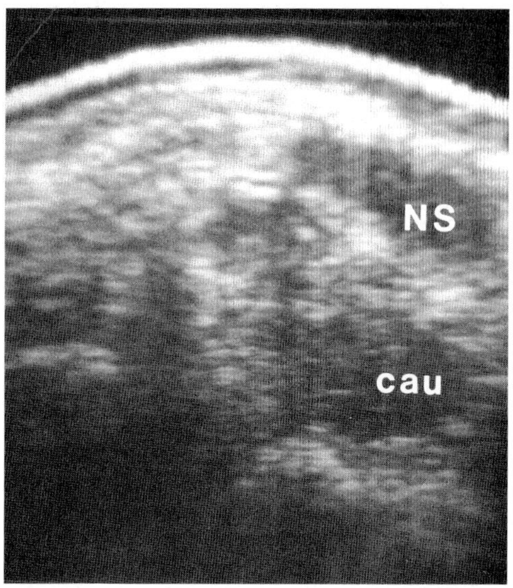

Fig. 51a. Acute hemorrhagic-necrotizing pancreatitis with areas of necrosis in tail and formation of a "necrotic pathway" into the anterior pararenal space on the left. cau = tail of pancreas; NS = necrotic pathway.

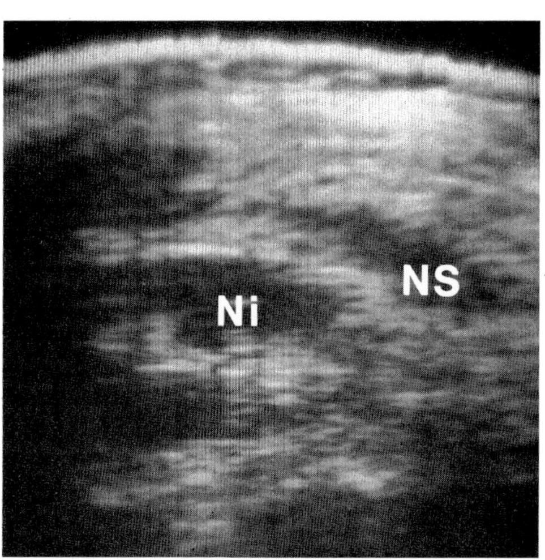

Fig. 51b. Acute hemorrhagic-necrotizing pancreatitis with areas of necrosis in tail and formation of a "necrotic pathway" into anterior pararenal space on left; same patient as in Fig. 51a. NS = necrotic pathway; Ni = kidney.

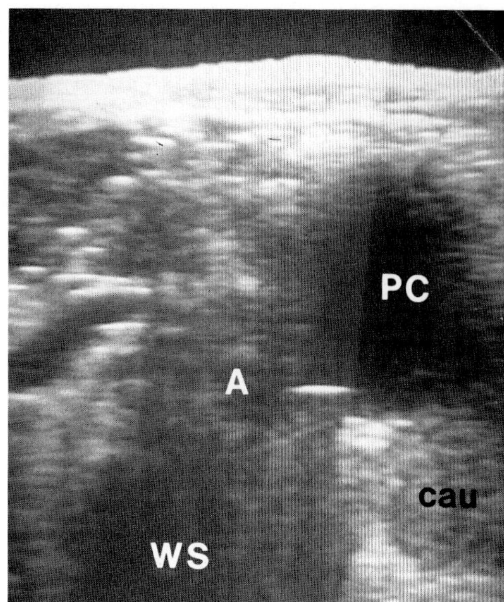

Fig. 52. Pancreatic pseudocyst at body/ tail interface in chronic relapsing pancreatitis (diameter about 6 cm). PC = pseudocyst; cau = tail of pancreas; A = aorta; WS = vertebral column.

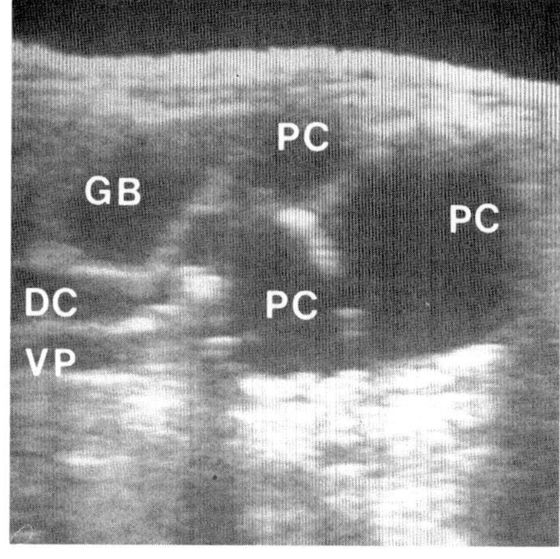

Fig. 53. Chronic relapsing (already calcified) pancreatitis with calcareous degeneration and pseudocysts. Distal choledochal stenosis induced by compression of common bile duct, with dilation of proximal duct segments. Included echo-rich areas, partly with dorsal sound elemination, correspond to pancreatic calcifications. PC = pseudocysts; GB = gallbladder (partly scanned); VP = portal vein; DC = common bile duct.

Abscesses, pleural effusions, pericardial effusions, fistulas, ascites, shock-induced renal alterations, and splenomegaly can likewise be uncovered by ultrasonography. The principal application of sonography is in following the disease course. It is an important aid in reaching a decision about surgical intervention [294, 339] (Table 21).

Beyond the acute disease, sonography of the upper abdomen is important for early diagnosis or developmental follow-up of pseudocysts, particularly with respect to determination of the need for surgery. The method allows the demonstration of changes in size and of consequences of a possible compression or displacement of adjacent organs (e.g., distal choledochal stenosis due to pseudocyst in region of pancreatic head with resultant congestion of prestenotic bile ducts (Fig. 53).

6.3 Diagnostic radiography

6.3.1 Conventional radiography

Conventional radiography is of limited applicability in acute pancreatitis and is used primarily to detect complications and to rule out other diseases (e.g., detection of free air in abdominal cavity with perforating ulcer). In some cases it also provides clues to the etiology (opacifying concrements) or, upon demonstration of pancreatic calcifications, to the presence of an acute attack of a chronic, calcified pancreatitis.

Plain films of the abdomen taken in upright or possibly also in lateral position can under some circumstances yield evidence of a generalized or circumscribed, usually paralytic ileus. Individual gas-filled, dilated small bowel loops in the left upper and medial abdomen ("sentinel loop"), and a sudden cessation of accumulation of intestinal gas in the region of the distal transverse colon, the left colonic flexure, or the descending colon (colon cutoff sign) are considered characteristic of, if not specific for, acute pancreatitis. In addition, overdistention of the duodenum and the proximal jejunum and an air-filled, atonic stomach are frequently observed, and less frequently diffuse "small-bowel levels" as signs of generalized ileus of the small intestine.

Plain chest x-rays, possibly supplemented by lateral films, fluoroscopy, or target-specific rotating radiography, can uncover pleural effusions, squamous atelectases, or pulmonary infiltrations.

Cholecystolithiasis detected by sonography and/or computed tomography requires no additional contrast radiography. When the bile ducts are obstructed at the same time, intravenous administration of a contrast medium for visualization of gallbladder and bile ducts has, moreover, little chance of success. Oral administration is not appropriate in this type of situation. It would, in addition, delay causal therapy. Sonographic or CT diagnosis of biliary reflux pancreatitis should therefore be followed immediately by an attempt at *endoscopic retrograde cholangiography* (ERC) with *endoscopic papillotomy* (EPT) (see Chapter 10). If an EPT cannot be carried out or fails for technical reasons, surgical intervention has to follow (see Chapter 11). In doubtful cases, a *percutaneous transhepatic cholangiography* (PTC) may contribute to differentiation of icterus caused by choledochal concretions from congestion due to pancreatic edema or pseudocysts, and confirm the need for surgery [143].

Angiographic study of the pancreas or upper abdominal organs is *not* indicated for the diagnosis of acute pancreatitis. Only in exceptional cases may it be used to help the surgeon to evaluate the vascular topography prior to surgery. However, *indirect splenoportography* is the method of choice for detection of splenic vein thrombosis and consequent segmental portal hypertension secondary to acute pancreatitis.

Contrast radiography of the gastrointestinal tract with barium sulfate is *contraindicated* during the acute illness. When the acute pancreatitis has subsided, an adjunctive small bowel series or barium enema is indicated only if stenoses or fistulas are suspected, inasmuch as pseudocysts are reliably detected by sonography and computed tomography.

In case an upper gastrointestinal hemorrhage is suspected, esophagogastroduodenoscopy is preferable to radiography. Besides a precise diagnosis, hemostasis by laser coagulation or sclerosing should be attempted concomitantly.

Pancreatic scintigraphy with ^{75}Se-methionine should *no longer* be performed in view of the radiation exposure and low sensitivity and specificity [62].

6.3.2   Computed tomography

Like sonography, computed tomography (CT), too, contributes to the discovery of etiological factors, to corroboration of the diagnosis, to evaluation of the severity and course of the disease, and to the detection of complications and associated diseases (Table 21). The two methods complement one another [144, 404]. Lackner et al. [261] have critically reviewed the advantages and disadvantages of the two techniques (Table 22).

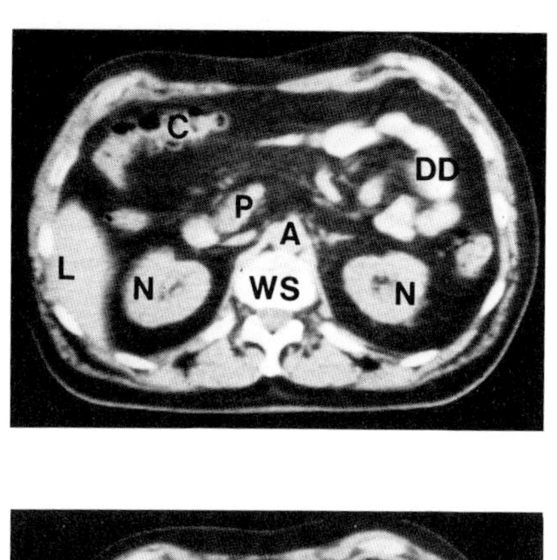

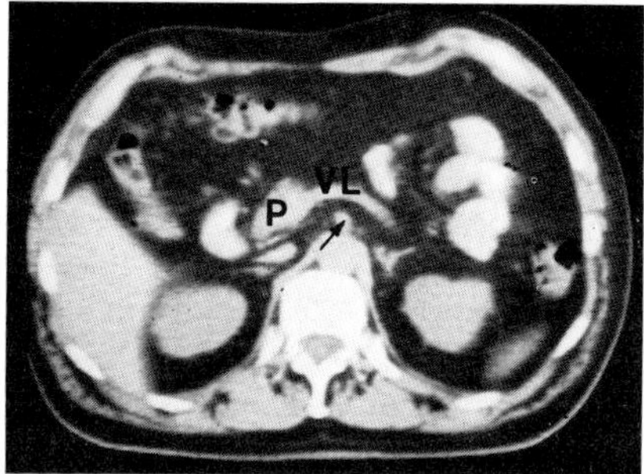

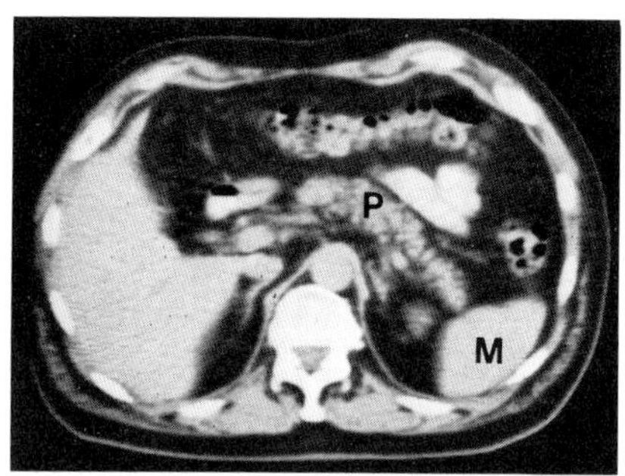

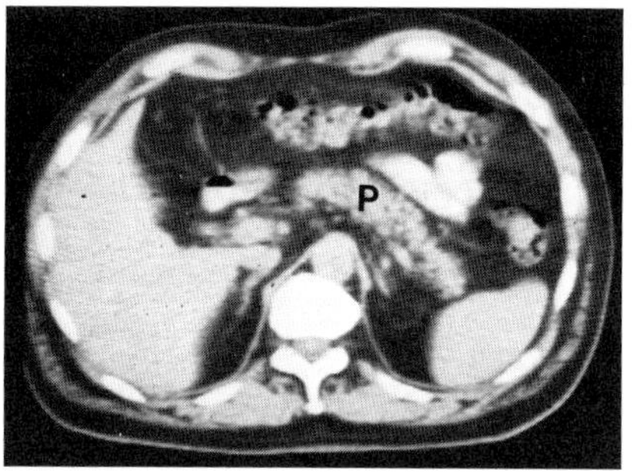

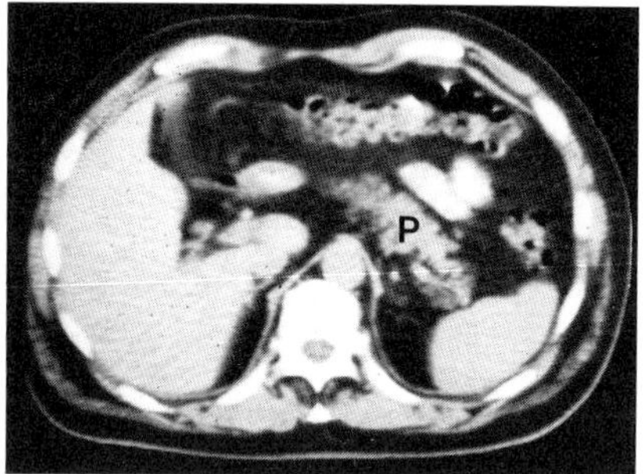

Figs. 54 a–e. Lobulated pancreas (normal computed tomography images). A = aorta; C = colon; DD = small bowel; L = liver; M = spleen; N = kidney; P = pancreas; VL = splenic vein; WS = vertebral column; → = superior mesenteric artery. (The computed tomograms and illustrations presented in Figs. 54–57 were supplied by courtesy of Prof. U. Scherer, M.D., Radiological Clinic, University of Munich; Director: Prof. J. Lissner, M.D.)

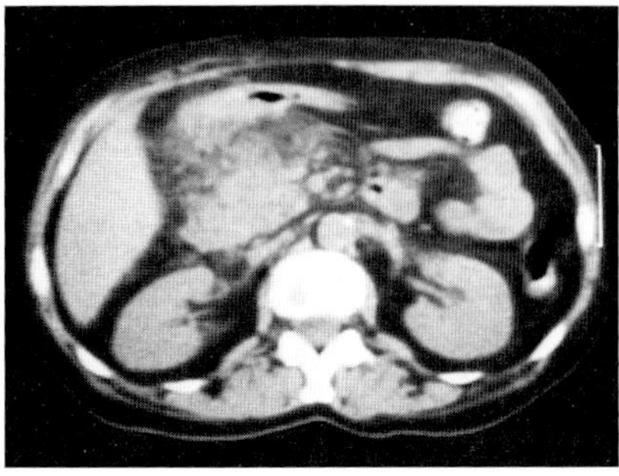 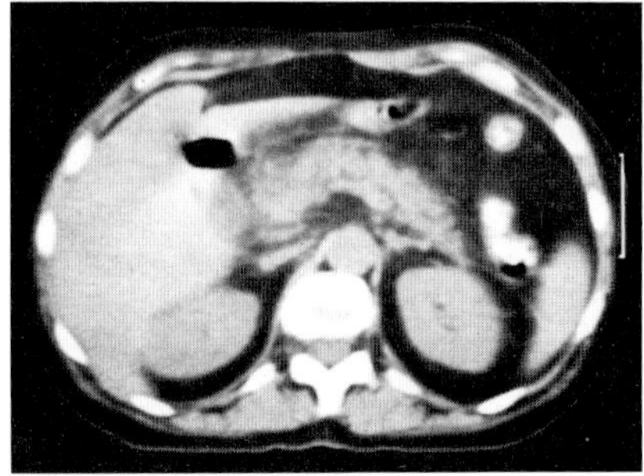

Figs. 55 a, b. Edematous pancreatitis (organ enlargement with unsharp outlines, particularly marked in region of pancreatic head).

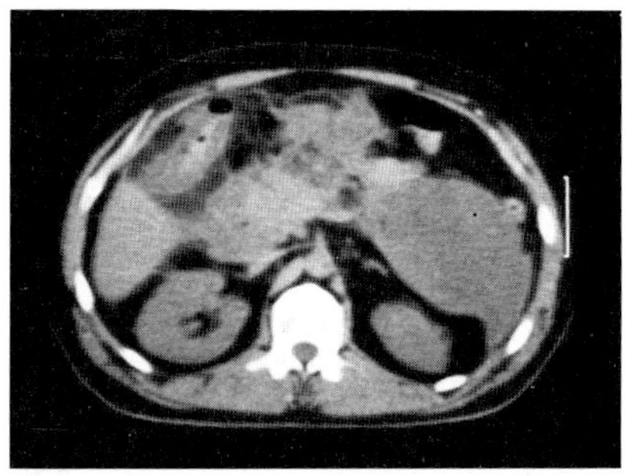

Fig. 56. Acute hemorrhagic-necrotizing pancreatitis (extensive necrosis in all segments of pancreas and spread of necrosis to bursa omentalis and anterior pararenal space left—"necrotic pathways" (see Chapter 8).

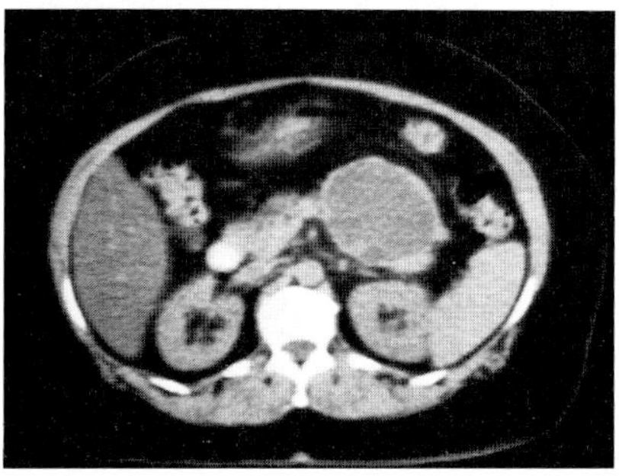

Fig. 57. Pancreatic pseudocyst in tail region (in chronic relapsing pancreatitis); alcoholic fatty liver as accessory finding.

The computed tomograms and illustrations were supplied by courtesy of Prof. U. Scherer, M.D., Radiological Clinic, University of Munich (Director: Prof. J. Lissner, M.D.).

Sonography, first of all, excludes other upper abdominal diseases and searches for a biliary origin. A "pancreatic edema" needs to be closely followed by sonography. If there is presumptive sonographic evidence of acute hemorrhagic-necrotizing pancreatitis and/or a severe clinical course, and particularly if surgical intervention is being considered, a CT study is indicated. The scope of the necrosis and its spread beyond the pancreas ("necrotic pathways") can be more readily determined by this means. On the basis of the CT findings, in turn, the patient needs to be closely monitored by sonography [339]. A detailed critical appraisal of the diagnostic value of the two methods, especially regarding their usefulness in establishing the need for surgery, has been presented by Neher et al. [339].

Figs. 54 a–e show normal CT images of the pancreas. An edematous pancreatitis appearing in the computed tomogram as organ enlargement with unsharp outlines, is depicted in Figs. 55 a, b. The morphological changes definable by computed tomography in acute hemorrhagic-necrotizing pancreatitis (areas of necrosis, necrotic pathways) are given in Fig. 56. Fig. 57 illustrates the detection of a pancreatic pseudocyst.

6.4   Diagnostic endoscopy

6.4.1   Esophagogastroduodenoscopy

Endoscopic examination of the esophagus, stomach and duodenum is not relevant to the primary diagnosis of acute pancreatitis. It is indicated, however, when hemorrhage from the upper gastrointestinal tract is suspected besides. It then serves to localize the source of the bleeding, such as a gastric or duodenal ulcer, for example, erosions, varices of the gastric fundus (in segmental portal hypertension due to splenic vein thrombosis), or esophageal varices (in concomitant alcoholic cirrhosis of the liver), and may be used therapeutically to stop the bleeding (Nd-YAG laser, sclerosing).

6.4.2   Endoscopic retrograde cholangiopancreatography (ERCP)

To perform ERCP is in general contraindicated in acute pancreatitis. However, retrograde cholangiography is necessary in the context of an endoscopic papillotomy (EPT) in biliary reflux pancreatitis (choledocholithiasis) (see Chapters 10, 11).

It should be noted in this connection that acute pancreatitis can develop in rare cases (also when there has been no prior pancreatic injury) following ERCP, particularly if parenchymal staining of the pancreas occurs as a result of unduly high injection pressure. Parenchymal staining should therefore be avoided at all costs. In the presence of pancreatic pseudocysts administration of the contrast medium can induce an infection of these cavities with ensuing abscess formation and sepsis. ERCP is therefore contraindicated in patients with pseudocysts except if the examination is performed immediately before a planned operation. Since these precautions began to be observed, acute pancreatitis induced by ERCP has occurred much less frequently than in the initial period of its use. Thus, Cotton [78] saw no further complications during his last 800 pancreaticographies.

6.4.3 Laparoscopy

In view of the available noninvasive morphological and clinical chemistry study methods, we consider it generally inadvisable to perform a laparoscopy to differentiate between edematous and hemorrhagic-necrotizing pancreatitis, as Arbeiter et al. [19] and Dagnini [86] have proposed. Lankisch [267] has further called attention to the fact that even under favorable conditions only a portion of the pancreas can be seen in laparoscopy. Consequently, the extent of organ destruction cannot be assessed, any more than the presence of abscesses or the course of necrotic pathways.

6.5 Adjunctive examinations

Among adjunctive examinations, we shall mention only the electrocardiogram (ECG) and electroencephalogram (EEG). As a rule, only uncharacteristic, general changes are found in the EEG in pancreatic encephalopathy, a possible, always threatening complication of acute hemorrhagic-necrotizing pancreatitis [238] (see Chapters 5 and 8). At the time of the patient's admission, the type of pain requires differential diagnosis to decide between acute pancreatitis and myocardial infarction (see Chapter 7). This differential diagnosis may be hampered by infarction-like ECG tracings sometimes observed in acute pancreatitis, which may be attributable to viscero-visceral reflexes or to direct myocardial damage from systemically active enzymes or toxic substances. Electrolyte shifts, too, can cause ECG changes in acute pancreatitis [238].

6.6 Studies after abatement of acute disease

Another search for possible causes of the acute pancreatitis should be undertaken once the acute symptoms have abated, if by that time the etiology of the illness remains uncertain [220]. In particular, studies that yielded no reliable data during the acute process (e.g., lipid status, Ca^{++}) ought to be repeated and supplemented and any etiological factors eliminated (e.g., clearing of bile ducts, removal of parathyroid adenomas, treatment of hyperlipoproteinemia). Persistent complications (e.g., pancreatic pseudocysts, diabetes mellitus) need to be ruled out.

The most important prognostic question, whether an acute pancreatitis or an acute attack of chronic pancreatitis has ended, is difficult to answer in many cases. The etiology provides some clues (biliary origin, chronic alcohol consumption). The existence of chronic pancreatitis is proved by evidence of pancreatic calcifications (pancreatolithiasis and parenchymal calcifications), but this evidence can be obtained only in an advanced disease stage, or by the discovery of persistent exocrine pancreatic insufficiency. This is demonstrated by pancreatic function tests with secretin and cholecystokinin or cerulein (to be done 3 months after abatement of pancreatitis at the earliest [82]). Chymotrypsin determination in the stool, the PABA-peptide test, and the fluorescein dilaurate test or radioimmunoassay of serum trypsin will detect only moderately severe or severe disturbances of exocrine pancreatic function so that pathological results, in contrast to pancreatic function tests, are obtained only in an advanced stage of the disease [354].

Chapter 7 – Differential Diagnosis

The diagnosis of acute pancreatitis not infrequently presents difficulties because the symptoms are often unclear and not very characteristic. The main reason for this is that the local inflammation can extend to neighboring organs so that the symptoms produced may actually be paradoxical.

The most important disease patterns to be considered in differential diagnosis are enumerated in Table 23.

Table 23. Differential diagnosis of acute pancreatitis

Intraabdominal disease processes	Extraabdominal-retroperitoneal disease processes
– Intestinal infarction	
– acute gallbladder-biliary tract disease: acute cholecystitis, cholecystocholedocholithiasis, cholangitis gallbladder perforation (gallbladder empyema)	– Myocardial infarction – Left-sided or right-sided renal or ureteral colic
– Perforating ulcer	
– Mechanical ileus	
– Rupture of aortic aneurysm	

Three groups of diseases in particular have to be ruled out in the differential diagnosis of acute pancreatitis. These are mesenteric infarction, myocardial infarction, and acute gallbladder-biliary tract diseases with or without an inflammatory component (cholangitis, cholecystitis, hydrops, empyema) and with or without obstructive jaundice.

7.1 Mesenteric infarction

Mesenteric infarction no doubt is the disease that most closely resembles acute pancreatitis in its objective and subjective effects: state of shock, severe impairment of general condition, causing the patient to feel "annihilated," and disturbed to absent intestinal activity. The painful sensations are similar, and abdominal palpation yields the same finding of pasty resistance.

Arterial mesenteric infarction does set in acutely but venous mesenteric infarction may be preceded by a prodromal phase of several days or, exceptionally, several weeks. It is characterized by mild abdominal pain and only slight disturbance of intestinal activity. Rectal examination occasionally produces blood on the finger. The manifestations are localized more in the left lower abdomen, a soft, pasty and relatively painless swelling being noted in the area of the small bowel loops predominantly affected by the infarction. The diagnosis can be made and corroborated by angiography.

7.2   Myocardial infarction

This differential diagnosis, too, is difficult because the ECG recorded in the acute phase of severe pancreatitis shows changes similar to those, and occasionally even typical for those, seen in myocardial infarction. Laboratory tests, sonography and, if necessary, computed tomography will, however, lead to the correct diagnosis. In rare cases there may actually be a true myocardial infarction at the same time. This is a situation which is most difficult and problematical in differential diagnosis (see Chapter 6).

7.3   Acute gallbladder and biliary tract diseases, complications

7.3.1   Acute cholecystitis

It is characterized by predominantly right-sided pain. This biliary pain usually lasts 2 or 3 hours, in contrast to the pain of pancreatitis, which extends over several days. On palpation, there is guarding in the right upper abdomen; at times a painful, inflamed gallbladder may be palpated (hydrops, empyema). Only in exceptional cases, however, does one also find icterus or subicterus with concomitant choledocholithiasis with or without cholangitis. At the same time the temperature is elevated and there is leukocytosis with leftward deviation, which is an uncommon finding in acute pancreatitis.

Specific laboratory tests, sonography and i.v. cholangiography and cholecystography will once again confirm the diagnosis, particularly in the simultaneous presence of a head pancreatitis or cholecystopancreatitis.

To be noted: The Courvoisier-Terrier syndrome involves a painless, congested, palpable gallbladder with jaundice! (Malignant obstructive jaundice, e.g., in carcinoma of pancreatic head.)

7.3.2   Perforation of gallbladder

In the initial phase the patient experiences the most severe pain, again in the right upper abdomen. Shortly thereafter there is considerable muscular defense of the abdominal wall and the general condition slowly worsens as a result of insidiously evolving biliary peritonitis. Extensive, now unmistakable peritonitis, with diffuse guarding of the entire abdomen, develops after a silent interval. This development and these symptoms are the exception in acute pancreatitis. The peritonitis is soon followed by subicterus of the sclerae with fever and guarding due to toxic absorption of the biliary perforation fluid.

7.3.3   Biliary peritonitis without perforation

A special form of gallbladder perforation is nonperforative biliary peritonitis due to pancreobiliary reflux into the gallbladder with secondary partial enzymatic digestion. In 1910, Clairmont and v. Haberer introduced the term for this special case of gallbladder perforation. The pathogenesis of this disease pattern remains controversial to this day.

On the other hand, every experienced abdominal surgeon is familiar with such gallbladder inflammations with the associated finding of a biliary exudate of the type seen in gallbladder perforation. Blad (1917) and Westphal (1929) came close to an explanation for this biliary peritonitis when they drew attention to the tryptic origin of this form of cholecystitis. The premise is that a mixture of pancreatic juice and bile, by pancreaticobiliary reflux via the cystic duct, makes possible the partial enzymatic digestion of the gallbladder wall with ensuing microperforation. Prolonged cholestasis and extended contact with the mucosa undoubtedly prepare the way. Accordingly, the principal pathogenetic factors are the disturbed blood flow through the congested gallbladder wall and the secondary partial enzymatic digestion due to pancreaticobiliary reflux into the gallbladder. This hypothesis is supported by the detection of amylase in the gallbladder [482].

7.3.4   Gallstone ileus

Another special case, and likewise a very dangerous complication of the complicated cholelithiasis, is the development of internal gallbladder or biliary tract fistulas, leading in extreme cases to *gallstone ileus*. For differential diagnosis, a plain film of the abdomen, as in perforating ulcer, supplies important and, if positive (presence of air), definitive evidence. Air in the biliary tract confirms the diagnosis and at the same time establishes the indication for repair or clearing of the biliary tree with cholecystectomy and removal of the fistula. Bilidigestive internal fistulas (internal communication between gallbladder or bile ducts and the stomach, duodenum, or colon) are extremely important for differential diagnosis because of the possibility of a "fitful" gallstone ileus, for aside from the ileus complication they can make the actual surgical procedure more difficult. Whenever possible, such patients should be operated on, at a reduced risk, before ileus develops.

7.4   Perforating ulcer

In these cases there is a boardlike rigidity extending from the upper to the lower abdomen, depending on the time course and the local perforative process. The detection of free air beneath the diaphragm on a plain film of the abdomen confirms the presumptive diagnosis. The air sickle phenomenon, however, is not present in all cases, as in covered perforation, for example. Absence of free air may not be taken as a basis for ruling out the presumptive diagnosis of perforating ulcer!

7.5   Renal colic

Colicky pain dominates this disease picture. A milder pain may simulate acute pancreatitis inasmuch as the process may be localized in the retroperitoneal space with radiation to the ureters. Palpation of the retroperitoneum (lumbar pain on percussion) and evaluation of the urine sediment in combination with sonography and intravenous urography are essential measures for establishing or revising the diagnosis.

7.6   Ileus due to small bowel strangulation or adhesions

A high ileus due to small bowel strangulation or adhesion with cramplike pains can also cause diagnostic confusion and difficulty. A markedly distended abdomen is noted with intestinal rigidity and severe impairment of the general condition (ileus intoxication), especially when ileus has been present for some time!

7.7   Aortic aneurysm

The covered rupture of an aortic aneurysm presents special diagnostic problems, particularly in overweight or obese patients. After a sudden onset the pattern of hemorrhagic shock with oliguria due to shock-induced renal insufficiency develops rapidly. Palpation reveals a pulsating abdominal mass of growing size and raises the suspicion of aortic aneurysm. Occasionally, an aneurysm is also detectable by the aortic thrill. This symptom, however, is present in only about one-half of the cases. Other indicative signs are the psoas phenomenon and absent crural pulses. The history includes bouts of abdominal pain radiating to the back, hypertension, or arteriosclerosis; less frequently, there are symptoms due to thromboembolism. However, pain is the cardinal symptom. It is of a cutting or lacerating type, in contrast to the pain in myocardial infarction, which has more of a crescendo character. Another important feature of the pain is its shift or migration, especially when retrosternal pain is experienced besides pain in the back and shoulders. The absence of repolarization defects in the ECG and of direct signs of infarction may aid in the differential diagnosis. Final clarification is achieved by sonography, which may be supplemented in doubtful cases by angiography or computed tomography. Rarely, the aneurysm will perforate the duodenum, with massive gastrointestinal hemorrhage resulting (Fig. 58).

Although not a very common disease, a dissective aortic aneurysm invariably calls for immediate surgery to prevent the patient from bleeding to death. Men of advanced age are affected most frequently, twice as frequently as women.

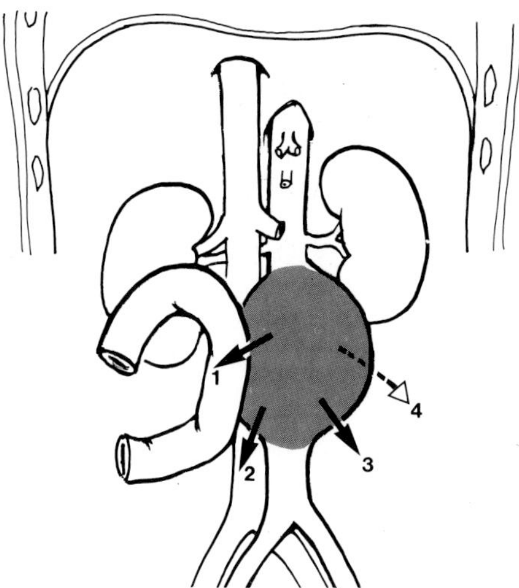

Fig. 58. Rupture of aortic aneurysm: 1, into the duodenojejunal flexure, which has been shifted to the right; 2, into lower vena cava; 3, into free abdominal cavity; 4, dorsalward into retroperitoneal space, the most common type. (From G. Carstensen, Arbeitsbuch Chirurgie, Urban & Schwarzenberg, 1982, p. 419.)

7.8 Acute abdomen induced by gynecological diseases, upper abdominal aneurysm

Finally, consideration must also be given in the differential diagnosis—apart from incarceration or angulation of the small intestine—to torsion of stalked organs in the lesser pelvis (ovarian cyst, omentum majus), to rupture of an ectopic pregnancy or, in the upper abdomen, to an aneurysm of the splenic artery.

7.9 Diagnostic peritoneal lavage

In problem cases diagnostic peritoneal lavage will be of help. This has to be performed in a technically refined and precise manner if sources of error and complications are to be excluded.

Method and technique:
This is the same as in peritoneal dialysis. In the midline, two fingerbreadths below the umbilicus, a stylet catheter is inserted through a stab incision after local anesthesia with epinephrine added, sterile precautions being observed (stylet catheter for peritoneal dialysis) (Fig. 59).

The bladder must first be emptied. The patient is in dorsal position. The drain with its perforated lower portion has to rest entirely inside the abdominal cavity. If bloody or cloudy fluid appears at once, the examination may be concluded once the specimen has been collected. If no fluid drains, the abdominal cavity is irrigated by infusion of isotonic saline solution. The lavage fluid is recovered by lowering the infusion bottle (siphonage, simply placing the infusion bottle on the floor).

In the case of less distinct macroscopic changes, a specimen of the fluid obtained is examined microscopically and biochemically (lipase, amylase).

Note:
In order to detect encapsulated or "trapped" accumulations of fluid or hematomas, it is necessary to advance the catheter in various directions while the patient is shifted to the lateral position.

Contraindications may arise after prior abdominal surgery and anticipated adhesions.

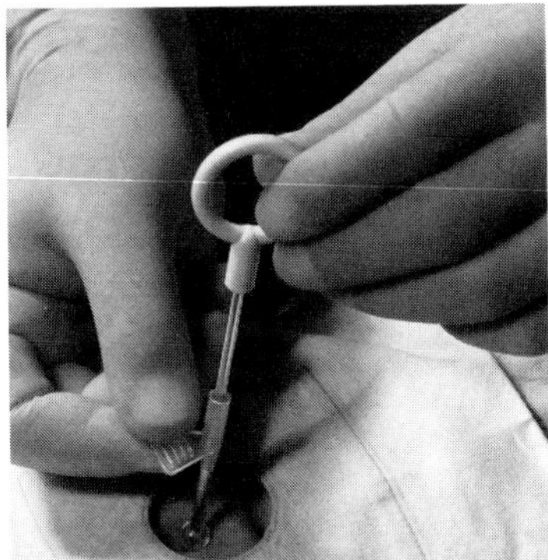
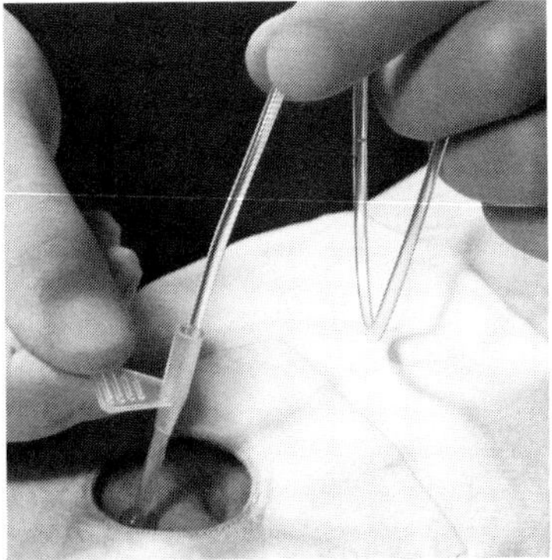
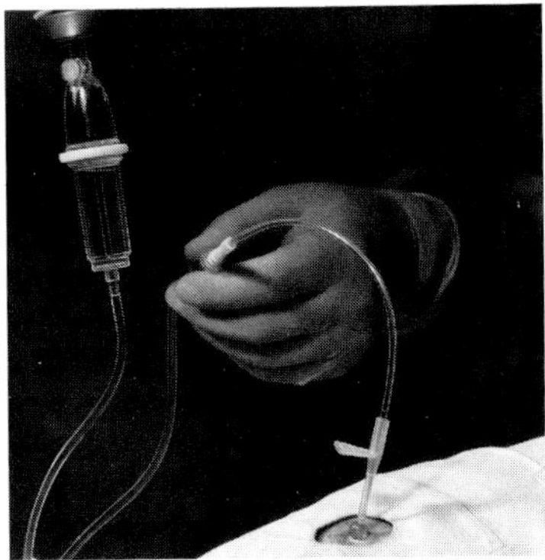

Fig. 59. (a) Indwelling plastic cannula; removal of trocar. (b) Introduction of catheter with closed, rounded tip. (c) Inflow of lavage fluid and diagnostic evaluation of refluxing irrigation fluid: strongly positive suspicion in case of macroscopically intransparent fluid. Microhemorrhages (independent of biochemical analysis for enzyme content) are detectable by microscopic examinations of sediment. (Peritofix kit, B. Braun Melsungen AG.)

There is a potential risk of injury to the tautly filled bladder or the intestine. Voiding of the bladder is an indispensable prerequisite! If there are surgical scars in the lower abdomen, the puncture should be made, if unavoidable, on the side of the scar or at a site remote from it.

A false positive result may be obtained because of bleeding from the puncture site. Such a misinterpretation can be avoided if attention is paid to the fact that only the infusion solution flowing back at the beginning shows bloody discoloration, whereas the solution draining later becomes clear (showing that the admixture of blood originated at the puncture site). For this reason epinephrine should be added to the local anesthetic for the puncture so that the oozing of blood from the stab wound may be prevented as far as possible. Another error causing a false positive result may be failure to advance the catheter to a sufficient depth in the abdominal cavity; blood from the stab wound may then pass through the perforations in the catheter into the lavage fluid and color it. A false result is also obtained if too little infusion fluid is used, since small or high accumulations may then escape irrigation.

Emergency laparoscopy may be locked upon as a competitive diagnostic procedure. This is a more demanding procedure and has to be performed by an experienced team of endoscopists (for diagnostic value, see Chapter 6, General and Special Diagnosis).

7.10   Posttraumatic pancreatitis following blunt abdominal trauma

Clinical features and symptomatology: The symptomatology of blunt pancreatic injuries in blunt abdominal trauma is variable and dependent in large measure on the scope of additional intraabdominal and extraabdominal injuries (multiple injuries!). In case of doubt, direct methods of examination, such as peritoneal lavage, have to be employed in lieu of indirect ones. Every obscure case requires additional recourse to angiography and, finally, to diagnostic, exploratory laparotomy.

Early symptoms, besides deep tenderness on palpation as noted in every case of acute pancreatitis, comprise slight rigidity of the upper abdomen due to the retroperitoneal encapsulation and occasional radiation of pain to the area between the two shoulder blades. It is important to take account of an early interval with a paucity of symptoms. This is attributable to the fact that small quantities of pancreatic secretion are initially tolerated and absorbed in the abdominal cavity, and that a developing peritonitis is at first confined to the bursa omentalis. Nausea and vomiting as well as the absence of intestinal peristalsis are side effects. Sonographic and radiographic examination of the abdomen (plain film) rarely yields abnormal findings at the outset or during the initial course. The plain x-ray is used, rather, to aid in the differential diagnosis and to detect serious associated complications such as duodenal rupture, biliary tract injury, and splenic or diaphragmatic rupture. The relative paucity of symptoms in the early stage should not blind us to the possibility of a fulminant disease course, which also exists in nontraumatic pancreatitis.

Accurate assessment of the disease is possible only by continuous interdisciplinary observation. Not infrequently, exploratory laparotomy or autopsy is required to uncover previously concealed pancreatic lesions or a posttraumatic pancreatitis following successful surgical treatment of combined injuries, such as splenic and hepatic rupture, which are more readily detectable because of massive bleeding.

Chapter 8 – Disease Course, Prognosis, and Complications

8.1 Prognosis

If an acute pancreatitis takes a generally serious course owing to local and general complications, this occurs less with the edematous variant than with the hemorrhagic-necrotizing disease form. The latter ends fatally in 35–85% of cases (see Chapter 11, Table 32).

By the same token, there is a correlation between the severity of an acute pancreatitis, hence its prognosis, and its etiological factors. Thus, the prognosis in biliary reflux pancreatitis – strictly speaking, the Opie syndrome – is poorer than it is in biliary non-canalicular or alcoholic pancreatitis.

Ranson and co-workers have described as prognostic indices 11 criteria which they rate as vital determinants (Table 24).

The prognosis worsens as the number of unfavorable parameters increases. These factors have to be completed by clinical manifestations, notably enzymatically induced encephalopathy (crises of agitation, mental confusion). This clinical phenomenon, however, must not be confused with a withdrawal delirium (delirium tremens) even though the two symptom constellations are similar and indicate a poor prognosis.

The general statement can be made that, from the clinical point of view, the prognosis of acute pancreatitis is determined by the onset or aggravation of a state of shock, persistence of ileus, development of renal and respiratory insufficiency (base deficit above 4 mmol/L, pO_2 below 60 mm Hg), a pancreatic encephalopathy, and gastrointestinal hemorrhages.

Table 24. Prognostically unfavorable parameters in acute pancreatitis (lethal factors according to Ranson et al. [373])

Initial/early findings	
Age	> 55 years
Serum glucose concentration	> 200 mg/dl
Leukocytosis	> 16,000/μl
LDH	> 350 U/l
SGOT	> 120 U/l
Subsequent findings (24–48 hr after onset of disease):	
Decrease of hematocrit	> 10%
Serum calcium concentration	< 2.0 mmol/l
Base deficit	> 4.0 mmol/l
Rise of blood urea nitrogen	> 5 mg/dl
Arterial pO_2	< 60 mm Hg
Fluid deficit	> 61

In terms of clinical chemistry, increases in WBC (leukocytosis in excess of $16,000\mu l$), serum glucose levels above 200 mg/dl, hypocalcemia of less than 2.0 mmol/l, decrease of hematocrit by more than 10% in the first 48 hours, increase of blood urea nitrogen by more than 5 mg/dl in the first 48 hours, and a rise of serum creatinine above 2.5 mg/dl are prognostically of crucial importance.

Guillemin recently reported on the phenomenon of nystagmus in patients with severe acute pancreatitis. Upon review, this proved to be the lethal factor in the majority of cases [200].

Lethality:
The lethality rate for acute pancreatitis varies according to its clinical course. While the hemorrhagic-necrotizing form (stages II to III) always has a high mortality rate, ranging up to 85%, mortality from edematous pancreatitis (stage I) is only 0−5%. As noted above, the etiology is the chief determinant of the mortality rate.

There are rare cases of hyperacute pancreatitis presenting a toxic clinical picture which causes death within a few short hours.

Clean described the case of a 23-year-old sailor who suddenly felt extremely severe abdominal pain while working in the engine room of his ship. He was dead 2 hours later! Autopsy uncovered hemorrhagic-necrotizing pancreatitis.

We made a similar observation in a secretary of age 19 who was referred to our clinic with cardiovascular collapse shortly after the sudden onset of very severe abdominal pain. She died 4 hours later. An acute hemorrhagic pancreatitis was found at autopsy.

Such cases which, according to statistics, account for 7% of all cases of acute pancreatitis, also pose a legal medical problem.

The spectrum of the causes of death depends largely on the disease course and on whether death occurred early or late (Tables 25, 26). Early deaths occur in the first 3 days after the onset of acute pancreatitis.

Wanke has listed the causes of death from acute pancreatitis in 94 men and 70 women included in a total of 15,107 autopsies (Table 27).

8.2 Complications

Numerous, manifold complications can develop in acute pancreatitis. They are summarized in Table 25.

Wanke has reported the following pathoanatomical findings based on a large number of autopsy case reports:

Table 25. Organ complications in acute pancreatitis*

Adipose tissue necrosis	158
peri-intrapancreatic	158
retroperitoneal	
subpleural	12
subepicardial	9
Necrotizing nephrosis	113
Acute damage to liver parenchyma	96
with jaundice	55
with hemorrhagic diathesis	27
Pleural effusions	76
Ascites	74
Hemorrhagic-erosive gastroduodenitis	44
Peritonitis	36
Stress ulcers	29
Myocardial infarction	27
Pericardial effusion	24
Portal vein thrombosis	12
Vascular erosions	11
(aorta, pancreaticoduodenal artery, splenic artery, splenic vein)	
Adrenal necrosis	9
Spontaneous splenic rupture	3

Table 26. Causes of death in 164 cases of acute pancreatitis (dependent on disease course, early/late lethality)*

Early lethality	*Late lethality*
Shock due to cardiac failure, 52%	infection (septic shock, abscess), 20%
due to respiratory failure (shock lung), 19%	hepatorenal insufficiency, 14%
	pulmonary embolism, 7%
	gastrointestinal hemorrhages due to: − vessel erosion, 8% − hemorrhagic diathesis, 5%

* Autopsy data from Pathological Institute, University of Heidelberg, and Municipal Hospital Rendsburg, Academic Hospital of the University of Kiel, 1963−1980; 164 cases among 15,107 autopsies.

Table 27. Causes of death in acute pancreatitis (164 cases among 15,107 autopsies)*

1. *Cardiac failure*	84
Postpancreatitic shock	67
Cardiogenic shock	17
2. *Infections*	33
Peritonitis	25
Postpancreatitic-septic shock	
Pneumonia	8
3. *Liver/kidney failure*	22
4. *Hemorrhages*	13
5. *Pulmonary embolism*	12

8.2.1 Shock

The most common complication is shock. However, different varieties of shock need to be considered. During the first few hours after the onset of an acute pancreatitis there is hypovolemic shock due to massive extra- and intracellular fluid loss resulting from permeability disorders caused by absorption of toxins and liberated kinins in the pancreatic area and retroperitoneal areas (see Chapter 6).

8.2.2 Renal failure

The second most frequent complication is renal failure, which is nearly always a direct consequence of shock or of toxic origin.

Oliguria or anuria may set in suddenly or develop slowly; occasionally, it disappears again, or it lasts for an extended period, or turns into chronic renal failure.

The pathogenetic mechanism of this renal complication is highly complex. It involves, besides the protracted shock, disturbances in water and electrolyte metabolism, intravascular coagulation, direct and indirect effects (kinins, histamine, toxic substances) on the kidneys by the enzymes released in the course of pancreatitis, sepsis, mechanical conditions due to retropancreatic hematoma and edema, and possibly associated reactions in the area of the aorticorenal autonomic nervous system.

Pathoanatomically, there usually is necrotizing nephrosis which in some cases also implicates the collecting tubule epithelia. Renal complications can occur in all stages and in all pathoanatomical forms of pancreatitis (shock-related parenchymal necrosis, septic nephritis, renal abscess). As a rule, they result from severe, extensive lesions produced by the autodigestive pancreatitis.

Bilateral adrenocortical necrosis is a comparatively rare complication.

8.2.3   Pleuropulmonary complications

Pleuropulmonary complications vary in degree of severity. The most serious form is acute respiratory insufficiency due to *shock lung* with severe hypoxemia. Other facotors, too, alone or in combination, that can lead to respiratory insufficiency are:
– retroperitoneal edema;
– elevation of diaphragm;
– left-sided and, at times, bilateral pleural effusion;
– pain-related restriction of abdominal respiration;
– bilateral basal pulmonary atelectases.

All these factors in conjunction with metabolic disorders cause tachypnea and an augmented oxygen deficit (see Chapter 3).

8.2.4   Hepatic insufficiency

Hepatic insufficiency can range from a simple subicterus to acute toxic hepatitis due to shock liver and effects of enzymes and toxic substances. In most cases the jaundice is caused by a disorder resulting from choledocholithiasis or cholangitis. However, it may also be due to compression of the retropancreatic or distal choledochus or to manifestations of intravascular hemolysis.

There have also been reports of sizable steatosis with the three components described by Wanke (the sequelae of portal enzyme derangement should be noted as well) and of diffuse forms of interstitial hepatitis.

Finally, mention should be made of necrotic foci and intrahepatic abscesses.

8.2.5   Local and extrapancreatic abscesses

These represent infection-induced complications. Such localized or diffuse single or multiple abscesses are due to superinfection of the pancreatitic foci of necrosis. The devascularized, necrotic tissue is an eminently suitable base for the development and multiplication of pathogenic microorganisms and so paves the way for superinfection. The abscesses seldom remain localized. They either lead to the formation of fistulas into a hollow organ or the free abdominal cavitiy, or they spread peripancreatically to the anatomically provided retroperitoneal septa.

This is how left-sided subphrenic and subhepatic abscesses or retrocolic abscess trails develop. Not infrequently, an abscess of the transverse mesocolon is observed. Retroperitoneal spread also reaches the renal bed and the iliac fossae as far as Douglas' space. Clinically, these abscesses generally occur between the 2nd and 13th weeks. They are accompanied by repeated attacks of septic fever, diffuse infiltration of the epigastrium, and severe worsening of the general condition, sometimes presenting the picture of septicemia or septic shock.

X-rays reveal the presence of retroperitoneal gas pockets. Sonography is more revealing, providing information about topography and scope and about the local pathway of the spread, thus helping to determine the optimal time for surgical intervention; this examination may be supplemented by computed tomography (see Chapter 6.3.2).

Considering the severity of the spontaneous development of these pancreatitis-related abscesses and resultant purulent liquefactions, surgical treatment for thorough removal of the contents and drainage of the abscesses is imperative. Extreme cases may require laparostomy ("open abdomen") treatment (see Chapter 11).

8.2.6 Fistulous complications in acute pancreatitis

External as well as internal fistulas can easily form after an operation or drainage.

8.2.6.1 External fistulas

8.2.6.1.1 *Pancreatic fistulas*
These develop in the area of the drainage channel or through the laparotomy wound, beginning on the 10th to 15th day. Fistula formation is heralded by an outflow of at first necrotic-purulent and later watery pancreatic secretion. Fistulas with small outflow volumes dry up in a short time owing to obliteration of the fistulous channel. Fistulas with large outflow volumes start at the head of the pancreas and are usually combined with a duodenal or biliary fistula. Their prognosis is unfavorable because they generate considerable water and electrolyte losses which are difficult to compensate. They are also the source of erosive complications, superinfections, and eviscerations (wound rupture).

8.2.6.1.2 *Gastrointestinal fistulas*
Gastric fistulas are recognizable by the fact that gastric juice and food remnants are discharged into the operative wound.

Duodenal fistulas result in death in the majority of cases. They are characterized by an extremely large secretion volume, which reaches several liters a day. The biliary, pancreatic, and intestinal components of the secretion have a severe macerating effect on all tissues and particularly the skin.

Intestinal fistulas (small and large bowel fistulas) likewise cause water and electrolyte losses that are difficult to offset.

Fistulas of the large intestine involve mainly the transverse colon and the left flexure of the colon. They can easily develop after the inadequate insertion of drains into the pancreatic compartment, resulting from colonic erosion. When feculent material is discharged from the drain, a pasty swelling of the operative field and the drainage tract is noted almost invariably. Not infrequently, death from these complications is preceded by sepsis with added colonic hemorrhage.

8.2.6.1.3 *Combined fistulas*
External fistulas of the pancreas and the digestive canal are often present at the same time. They originate from a pancreatic focus of suppuration which has liquefied between the pancreatic compartment, the stomach, colon and duodenum; they also develop in connection with the drains inserted in the first operation and their exit channel through the abdominal wall.

8.2.6.2 Internal fistulas

8.2.6.2.1 *Pancreatodigestive fistulas*
These discharge necrotic material from the autodigestive pancreatitic process into the large intestine, stomach, duodenum, the remaining small intestine or the biliary tract.

8.2.6.2.2 *Internal colonic fistulas*

These generally form between the 4th and 8th weeks of the illness. They are detected by disturbed transit associated with subicterus or diarrhea. Their suspected presence can be confirmed by filling the fistulous tract with contrast medium or by barium enema. However, such an examination is indicated only in the postacute stage. If it should prove necessary earlier, the use of a water-soluble (!) contrast medium is advisable so that the threatening development of a barium peritonitis due to escape of barium-containing contrast medium into the abdominal cavity may be avoided.

Colonic fistulas develop in the presence of a mesocolic or mesenteric abscess.

8.2.6.2.3 *Gastric fistulas*

These very frequently necessitate a supplementary, added operation to prevent retention and superinfection.

8.2.6.2.4 *Duodenal fistulas*

Such fistulas are due to abscesses in the head of the pancreas. They may therefore be associated on occasion with severe bleeding from the digestive canal, which requires immediate intervention.

8.2.6.2.5 *Fistula formation in bile ducts*

Fistulas rarely form in the bile ducts. They are caused by necrosis of the duodenum and necrosis of the terminal choledochus.

8.2.6.2.6 *Communicating fistulas*

Finally, complex foxhole-like communicating fistulas may develop between several organs.

8.2.7 Hemorrhagic complications

Numerous causes of these complications can be cited. Clinically, they present three aspects:

8.2.7.1 Intraabdominal hemorrhages

These are detectable by bleeding from drains or drainage channels or from the laparotomy wound. They are due to erosion of the peripancreatic vessels and, less commonly, the celiac trunk, the gastroduodenal artery and, exceptionally, of the superior mesenteric artery. The prognosis of these hemorrhages is always very unfavorable. The lethalitiy rate exceeds 80%.

8.2.7.2 Hemorrhages due to coagulation disorders

Such hemorrhages occur mainly from the 12th to 25th day of illness on. They result either from a disorder of hepatic synthesis (e.g., hypoprothrombinemia) or from an intravascular coagulation defect leading to consumption coagulopathy. Occasionally, the exact etiological factor is not discernible. The therapeutic possibilities are sharply restricted as a consequence. There may also be a toxic or enzymatic bone marrow lesion produced by the direct or indirect effects of the enzymes released during the pancreatitis.

8.2.7.3   Gastrointestinal hemorrhages

(Bleeding of fundus varices, due to segmental portal hypertension, erosive gastroduodenitis, stress ulcers, Mallory-Weiss syndrome.) They are a prognostically unfavorable sign and frequently sequelae of septicemia and paralytic ileus (Table 28).

8.2.8   Necroses and perforations

8.2.8.1   Intestinal wall lesions

Concomitantly with the hemodynamic effects, intestinal edema or intestinal wall lesions due to intramural enzyme action may be produced. It is by this route that colonic, duodenal, or gastric necrosis develops in the course of a pancreatitis. Such complications involving direct intramural enzyme action or enzyme action along the retrocolic necrotic pathways, which end fatally in 4 out of 5 cases, are fortunately rare. However, symptoms of local peritonitis always necessitate surgical intervention (see 8.2.5).

Punctiform or segmental areas of necrosis and small bowel perforations are traceable to circulatory disturbances such as a shock-induced blood flow deficit in the intestinal wall in conjunction with the extrapancreatic effect of the autodigestive process, or with direct autodigestion of the intestinal wall. The clinical syndrome is that of a generalized acute peritonitis. This finding, too, calls for surgical intervention, to wit, diagnostic-exploratory laparotomy.

Table 28. Clinical complications of acute pancreatitis

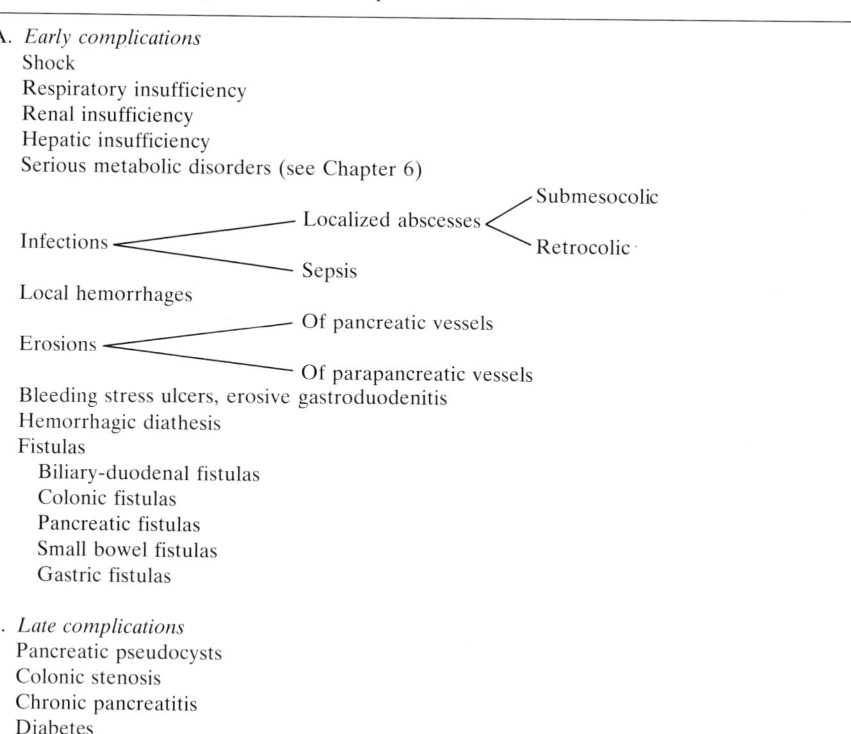

A. *Early complications*
   Shock
   Respiratory insufficiency
   Renal insufficiency
   Hepatic insufficiency
   Serious metabolic disorders (see Chapter 6)

   Infections — Localized abscesses — Submesocolic / Retrocolic
   Infections — Sepsis
   Local hemorrhages

   Erosions — Of pancreatic vessels
   Erosions — Of parapancreatic vessels
   Bleeding stress ulcers, erosive gastroduodenitis
   Hemorrhagic diathesis
   Fistulas
      Biliary-duodenal fistulas
      Colonic fistulas
      Pancreatic fistulas
      Small bowel fistulas
      Gastric fistulas

B. *Late complications*
   Pancreatic pseudocysts
   Colonic stenosis
   Chronic pancreatitis
   Diabetes

8.2.8.2 Necrosis and perforation of bile ducts

These represent a rare but severe complication of acute pancreatitis. They are detectable by the development of biliary peritonitis. Laparotomy reveals choleperitoneum. Two pathogenetic mechanisms are implicated: the proteolytic enzymatic effect on the choledochal wall, or thrombosis of a small choledochal artery with secondary necrosis. The disease is associated with paralytic ileus. Follow-up examinations by plain films of the abdomen are always necessary for this reason.

8.2.9 Splenic complications

Thrombosis of the splenic vein due to further expansion of the pancreatic edema or pancreatic necrosis, secondary peripancreatic fibrosis, or a pseudocyst can lead to segmental, peripheral portal hypertension and the development of fundal and, in the further course, esophageal varices. In the extreme case, this in turn results in severe gastrointestinal variceal bleeding. In such cases splenectomy offers the possibility of a cure. Also to be noted is the possibility of splenic infarction, intrasplenic hematomas, and spontaneous splenic rupture due to enzymatic destruction of the capsule.

8.2.10 Pancreatic pseudocysts

Postacute pancreatic pseudocysts (see Chapter 11).
When there is a considerable mass of necrotic detritus, it cannot be completely absorbed. The result is encapsulation of the focus, which transforms into a pseudocyst. This takes place in two phases:

In the initial phase a mixture of necrotic debris, blood, and enzyme-containing secreta accumulates in the pancreatic region. If this remains sterile, a pseudocyst gradually forms. This necrotic-hemorrhagic exudate is encapsulated by the neighboring organs. Once the necrotic tissue and the blood have been enzymatically liquefied, the pseudocyst manifests itself through mechanical displacement (Fig. 60). Pseudocysts can undergo spontaneous remission within weeks.

The frequency with which pseudocysts have been seen in the last 10 years must surely be viewed in relation to the therapeutic effectiveness of intensive medical care. The patients tend to experience more locally controlled disease processes of this type. The pseudocyst generally becomes clinically apparent through the effects of displacement, either by pyloroduodenal compression with stenosis, compression of the bile duct, a perforation, fistula, or hemorrhage due to ulceration of a large vessel, or by development of a large, palpably resistant tumor. Sonography of the abdomen also frequently uncovers smaller pseudocysts. The pseudocyst development may involve the stomach wall or the mesocolon, compromising wall perfusion, and formation of an internal scar with ulceration. Pseudopyloric scars thus form in many cases.

Compressions with stenosis are rare complications. According to past experience, they occur in the upper abdomen as a result of displacement. When localized in the lower abdomen and lower intestinal area, they point to a suppurative focus in the retrocolic regions.

Late sequelae of pancreatic trauma. These consist of posttraumatic pancreatic fistulas and the development of posttraumatic pseudocysts. Not infrequently, too, pancreatic injuries that took an uncomplicated course are detected several months later by the formation of a pseudocyst; this occurs in about 20% of all cases. The pathogenetic precondition for a pseudocyst is either a prior duct lesion or prior pancreatitis.

Topographically, there are several possible variants of cyst development: intrapancreatic, extrapancreatic-retroperitoneal, and extrapancreatic-intraperitoneal-parapancreatic (Fig. 60).

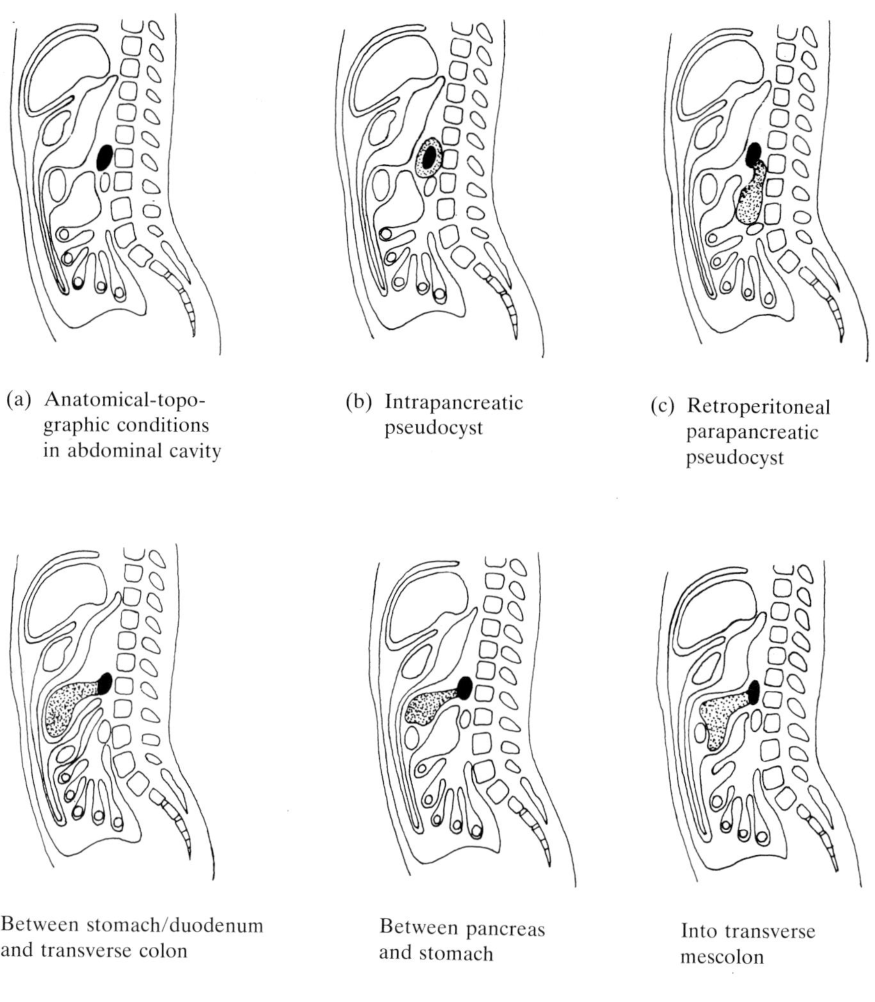

Fig. 60. Possible developments and directions of expansion of posttraumatic pancreatic pseudocysts and resultant organ displacements [335].

8.2.11   Colonic stenoses

These have been observed in the late disease course. They result from fibrous constriction, vascular thrombosis, or retrocolic accumulation of exudate with ensuing abscess formation. On occasion they heal spontaneously. They have to be differentiated from a neoplastic process with tumorous stenosis. Colonoscopy or, if this is not possible, a cautious barium enema will establish the differential diagnosis.

8.2.12   Chronic calcifying pancreatitis

Mention should finally be made of evolving chronic calcifying pancreatitis in the later course, marked by calcific deposits in the parenchyma or in the pancreatic duct system, also called calcified pancreatitis or pancreatolithiasis. This complication occurs at a rate of 10–15%. It should always be borne in mind that chronic pancreatitis may have preceded an acute pancreatitic attack.

8.2.13   Permanent diabetes

Permanent diabetes is a classic late complication of acute pancreatitis that is caused by destruction or fibrosis of the glandular parenchyma in the body-tail region. This incretory pancreatic insufficiency occurs in 2–10% of all cases of pancreatitis and should not be mistaken for tansitory hyperglycemia during the acute disease process. Some reports of higher incidence rates are based on inadequate differentiation.

Chapter 9 – General Aspects
of Current Pancreatitis Therapy

At the beginning of this century the treatment of acute pancreatitis was predominantly surgical. From our present vantage point this approach was bound to yield unfavorable results and, consequently, to bring on a changeover to completely conservative therapy because the pathomorphogenetic and pathophysiological processes involved in acute pancreatitis and its complications, with their specific, almost invariably shock-promoting mechanisms, were not sufficiently well known at that time.

The general, intensive-care background therapy has thus been significantly complemented by special therapeutic modalities based on pathogenetic as well as pathophysiological discoveries. These include, e.g., the elimination of etiological factors, early use of protease inhibitors, "deactivation" of the gland, and clearing the body of enzymes, kinins, and toxic substances.

Advances have also been achieved in terms of optimized diagnostic procedures such as intensive monitoring, sonography, and computed tomography for the indispensable developmental control.

If remote toxic and circulatory effects arising from the local autodigestive inflammatory process, hence the critical causative condition determining the prognosis, persists, conservative treatment alone, which cannot control the local inflammation, will not produce a curative effect, either. Presumably owing to skepticism concerning renewed attempts at surgical treatment, the idea of an active conservative-surgical approach in acute hemorrhagic-necrotizing pancreatitis – including early therapeutic laparotomy – has been prematurely dismissed. The important points at issue are not alone improved operative techniques but also the need to prevent or interrupt local effects of the disease. Although formerly considered difficult to operate on, the pancreas is today no longer under the "noli me tangere" ban.

Optimal intensive conservative therapy and surgical intervention should not be considered as competitive but should be weighed from case to case as mutually complementary therapeutic measures. In problematic or doubtful cases surgical intervention is not only debatable but often unavoidable. Removal of a prepapillary concretion in particular–insofar as this cannot be done endoscopically–is a "conditio sine qua non" in biliary reflux pancreatitis from the pathomorphogenetic and pathophysiological viewpoint, respectively.

The concept of interdisciplinary conservative-active therapy is based on the solid knowledge and experience gained in intensive medical care. If the patient's general condition deteriorates in spite of optimal conservative treatment, timely laparotomy not only permits direct inspection of the local changes but makes it possible to follow through therapeutically by proceeding to a target-specific surgical correction of the pancreatitic process. The degree of risk and the optimal timing of the operation will dictate the therapeutic action and, in the final analysis, determine the prognosis of this invariably grave and forever problematical gastroenterological disease.

Chapter 10 – Conservative Therapy of Acute Pancreatitis

The therapeutic approach to acute pancreatitis–aside from general, basic therapy comprising parenteral fluid and electrolyte replacement, no food or fluids being given by mouth, and pain control–has to be guided by the etiology, severity, and progress of the disease. The extremely difficult and vital decision whether to operate and when should be made jointly by all the specialists participating in the intensive care. In every case of acute pancreatitis, therefore, and also in severe attacks of chronic relapsing pancreatitis, diagnosis should be followed immediately, if at all possible, by interdisciplinary surveillance and treatment so that the internist and the surgeon can jointly follow the clinical course.

There is as yet no universally accepted therapeutic concept. A broad consensus exists only with respect to basic therapy. Specific therapeutic modalities are based on pathophysiological findings (Fig. 61) (see also Chapter 3). They include measures to inhibit the exocrine pancreatic secretion designed to achieve a reduction of secretory pressure in the pancreatic duct system and of enzyme parapedesis and, consequently, a lessening of autodigestion and of the rate of complications.

An attempt is also made to influence the autodigestion directly by administering enzyme inhibitors, for the effectiveness of which there is experimental evidence. Besides aprotinin (Trasylol®), the most widely tested protease inhibitor, other protease inhibitors, and phospholipase inhibitors, therapeutic peritoneal lavage has also been proposed for the treatment of acute pancreatitis (elimination of enzymes, kinins, and topic substances).

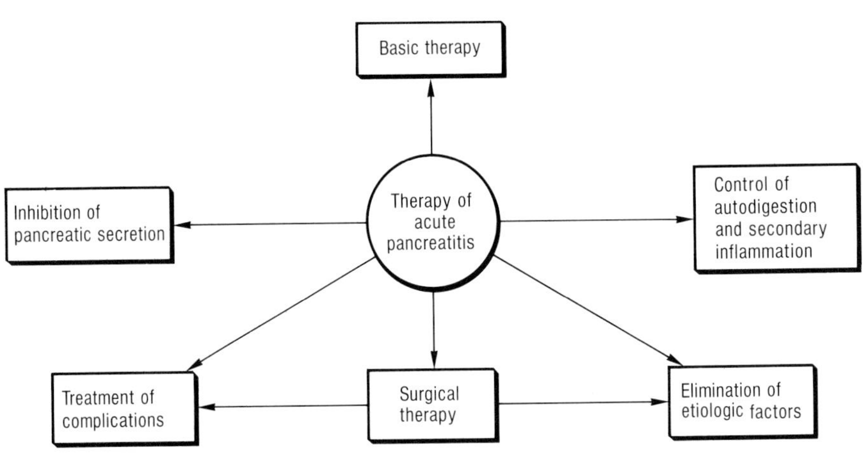

Fig. 61. Therapeutic approaches to acute pancreatitis

A causal therapy to interrupt the pathophysiological mechanism of the disease (e.g., removal of a prepapillary choledochal stone) is particularly desirable. Prevention as well as early detection and treatment of complications presuppose intensive monitoring of the diesease course.

10.1   Pain control

The symptom of acute pancreatitis that causes the patient the most distress is pain. Pain relief is therefore one of the first therapeutic requirements. This also serves to deactivate the gland, since the pain can provoke a central stimulation of pancreatic secretion [103, 143]. In addition, it stops the harmful effect of pain on blood flow, particularly in the pancreas and the myocardium (reflex vasoconstriction) [9, 406].

Morphine is contraindicated in acute pancreatitis because of its action in contracting the sphincter of Oddi [128]. Since morphine derivatives (e.g., pethidine, meperidine) can also increase sphincter tone, if to a lesser degree, they should not be employed as analgesics of first choice. Many authors recommend procaine hydrochloride (up to 2 g/24 hr) [156]. At this dose level cardiac side effects (AV-block) generally do not occur. However, there have been warnings about a possible anaphylactic reaction [170]. Inasmuch as antispasmodics can have a shock-enhancing effect, their use is controversial [51]. When administering analgesics, it should be borne in mind that many of them affect coagulation and can be ulcerogenic. For these reasons we recommend pentazocine (Fortral®) as analgesic in acute pancreatitis. A possible pain-relieving effect of glucose and insulin infusion is discussed under 10.2.3. The aspiration of gastric secretions is said to relieve pain through decompression. Drugs that are used in the treatment of acute pancreatitis because of their antisecretory effect on the exocrine pancreas (e.g., anticholinergics, calcitonin; see 10.3) are also said to alleviate the pain. A similar effect has been observed after the administration of protease inhibitors (aprotinin, Trasylol®) (see 10.4).

Surgeons in particular have recommended epidural analgesia as well as infiltration of the splanchnic nerve or the ligamentum teres with local anesthetics in very severely painful states that do not respond to the aforementioned measures [143, 195, 503]. Besides an analgesic effect, an improvement of the microcirculation has been reported to result [143].

10.2   Basic therapy

The basic therapy of acute pancreatitis, which includes the measures for pain control described above, is summarized in Table 29. An information about the surveillance of patients with acute pancreatitis is being presented first inasmuch as important therapeutic conclusions can be drawn from this findings.

Table 29. Basic therapy in acute pancreatitis

- Pain control: e.g., pentazocine, procaine hydrochloride; beware of morphine! (increases tone of sphincter of Oddi)
- Intensive monitoring (Table 30)
- No food or fluids by mouth ("deactivation of pancreas"); in addition, gastric aspiration in ileus or subileus
- Parenteral volume and electrolyte replacement (correction of balance! Check central venous pressure!)
- Infusion of glucose (blood sugar tests; depending on blood sugar levels, i.v. infusion [Perfusor!] of regular insulin [unmodified insulin]), glucose substitutes, and amino acids; also, in further course, infusions of lipid solutions for parenteral nutrition in patients having no major disturbances of fat metabolism
- Supplementation of human albumin at reduced serum albumin levels and in shock; blood transfusions in case of reduced hemoglobin and hematocrit

---

10.2.1 Surveillance of patients

The patient needs to be closely monitored even with an apparently innocuous onset of disease (Table 30). Blood pressure, pulse, and urine excretion should be checked hourly so that shock or incipient renal failure may be detected and treated early. If hypovolemic shock is suspected, recording of central venous pressure (CVP) provides additional information, as also in case of excessive fluid administration or concomitant cardiac failure (beware of pulmonary edema!). The fluid balance should be calculated every 6–12 hours.

Blood sugar tests (every 6 hours or so) can detect metabolic or iatrogenic hyperglycemia in time (see 10.2.3 and 10.6.4). Depending on the severity of the illness, the serum electrolytes, hematocrit and hemoglobin, WBC, arterial pO_2 and pCO_2, and the acid-base metabolism should be regularly checked about every 6, 12, or 24 hours. Serum lipase (or amylase), creatinine, BUN, coagulation tests, total protein, albumin, bilirubin, LDH, γ-GT, and transaminases have to be monitored daily, and cholesterol and triglycerides should be kept in mind. Determination of methemalbumin is said to be helpful for evaluation of the clinical course [273] and so is determination of phospholipase A_2 [420] (see 6.1.1.2).

A clinical examination should be carried out at least twice a day, special attention being paid to signs of ileus or subileus, ascites, pseudocysts, and pleural effusions, and to pulmonary and cerebral symptoms. The sonographic examination can uncover changes in the size of the pancreas, changes in organ structure (e.g., necrosis), necrotic pathways, abscess formation, pseudocysts, ascites, or pleural effusions as well as pathological changes of the gallbladder (e.g., cholecystolithiasis, cholecystitis, or hydrops) and biliary tract (congestion, choledocholithiasis). Radiography may confirm, a clinically suspected ileus (plain film of abdomen). Pulmonary infiltrations or pleural effusions are demonstrable by chest x-rays. Developmental ECG control is necessary not only for differential diagnosis but also for timely detection of myocardial complications (see Chapter 6).

Table 30. Parameters for surveillance of patients with acute pancreatitis (see Chapter 6)

- Blood pressure, pulse, central venous pressure, urine excretion, fluid balance (edema, exudate, pseudocyst fluid, etc. to be considered!), temperature
- Electrolytes (Na^+, K^+, Ca^{++}, phosphate), CBC, glucose, lipase, α-amylase, coagulation status, creatinine, BUN, total protein, albumin, γ-GT, alkaline phosphatase, transaminases, bilirubin, LDH, lipids, arterial pO_2, pCO_2, acid-base metabolism, possibly methemalbumin, phospholipase A_2
- Clinical examination, particularly local changes, intestinal motility, ascites, pseudocysts, pleural effusion, pulmonary and cerebral complications
- Sonography, possibly computed tomography: edema, necrosis, necrotic pathways, abscess, pseudocysts, ascites, biliary tract, liver, spleen, pleural effusion
- Radiography: chest (pleural effusion, pulmonary infiltration), abdomen (intraluminal gas distribution, e.g., sentinel loop, colon cutoff signs)
- ECG

10.2.2 Ban on oral feeding

The ban on oral food and fluid intake serves to "deactivate the gland." It is also meant to avert exacerbation of an existing subileus or ileus, not to mention worsening of the patient's subjective symptoms (pain, nausea, vomiting) following food intake.

There are doubts about the usefulness of a nasogastric tube as part of standard therapy. It was not found to have a positive effect in the treatment of mild or moderately severe pancreatitis [139, 285]. However, a nasogastric tube is indispensable in severe cases, particularly in the presence of symptoms of subileus or ileus.

10.2.3 Parenteral replacement of fluid, electrolytes, nutrient solutions, albumin, and blood

Immediate, adequate replacement of fluids and electrolytes is probably the most important of the therapeutic measures. The required volumes ought not to be underestimated since the circulation may be deprived of several liters by pancreatic edema, vasodilation in the splanchnic region, ileus, ascites, vomiting, or aspiration of gastric secretion. This has to be taken into account in correcting the fluid balance. Attention has been called above to the importance of checking CVP. Electrolyte supplementation will depend on the measured serum levels. Hypocalcemia, as a prognostically unfavorable parameter, should be watched for as carefully as hypokalemia and hypophosphatemia. In addition, human albumin and transfusions may have to be given in shock and hemorrhages.

To counteract a catabolic metabolism, parenteral alimentation should be started early. Glucose, glucose substitutes, and amino acids should be given to begin with 30 kalories per kg daily, these amounts to be carefully increased to 60 kalories per kg daily by added parenteral administration of lipid solutions if there are no major disturbances of the fat metabolism [143]. The infusion of glucose should be accompanied by measurements of blood sugar and, commensurately to the blood sugar values, by simultaneous i.v. infusion (Perfusor!) of regular insulin (unmodified insulin). Inasmuch as parenteral administration of calories can provoke a stimulation, though slight, of exocrine pancreatic secretion [246] it has been the subject of controversy, particularly as far as the use of fat solutions is concerned. However, during a protracted disease course it is indispensable [269].

Some authors have reported relief of pain being accomplished by simultaneous infusion of glucose and insulin. This effect is said to be due to inhibition of the adipose tissue lipase and, consequently, reduction of adipose tissue necrosis [179, 445]. Yet, since the effect was statistically significant only in the first 24 hours, doubts have been expressed about the efficacy of this step [51, 103].

10.3 Inhibition of pancreatic secretion

Most important for reducing the activity of the gland is abstinence from food and fluid intake. On the other hand, some authors have recommended antacids for buffering gastric acid and thus preventing the release of secretin in the duodenum. However, systematic antacid treatment requires continuous administration of sizable volumes by mouth. This conflicts with the first therapeutic rule of deactivation and ileus therapy. We therefore disapprove of it. Occasional administration of antacids is of no use to begin with.

The administration of acid secretion blockers, such as cimetidine or anticholinergics, may be considered, however. Yet no improvement of the disease course has been observed, either experimentally [112] or clinically [377], following the use of cimetidine. With regard to cimetidine (Tagamet®) therapy it should also be noted that four cases of acute pancreatitis coinciding with cimetidine treatment have been reported in the meantime [22, 205] (see Chapter 2). No causal relationship has been demonstrable so far. Ranitidine, a new H_2-blocker (Sostril®, Zantic®), may be also applied.

Also to be weighed in this connection is use of the anticholinergic pirenzepine (Gastrozepin®), which acts mainly on the stomach. Broadly effective anticholinergics such as atropine, for example, inhibit pancreatic secretion not only indirectly, through reduction of gastric acid, but directly as well. Yet their use cannot be recommended because of undesirable side effects, such as exacerbation of subileus, ileus, or shock [269]. Moreover, no advantageous effect was seen in a controlled study [68].

Substances that find application in the treatment of acute pancreatitis because of their inhibitory effect on exocrine pancreatic secretion are listed in Table 31. Inasmuch as carbonic anhydrase blockers (acetazolamide, Diamox®) only depress the hydrokinetic function of the pancreas but do not affect the ecbolic one, they are unacceptable, generally speaking, because of the danger of thickening of pancreatic secretions and because of their side effects [238].

Glucagon does reduce exocrine pancreatic secretion as well as gastric secretion but, according to controlled studies, has no positive effect on lethality or the course of acute pancreatitis [106, 256]. This statement should be qualified, however, by noting that the general lethality rate in these studies was low.

According to two double-blind trials [157, 359] calcitonin, which inhibits the ecbolic pancreatic secretion and gastric secretion, has a beneficial effect on the clinical course although it does not lower the lethality rate in acute pancreatitis. This was not confirmed, however, in another controlled clinical study [509].

There have been conflicting reports about the effect of somatostatin in experimental pancreatitis [274, 424]. Positive trends noted in preliminary studies with a small number of patients [288, 462] require corroboration by controlled trials. A multicenter study of this type is in progress at the present time [461].

In view of the generally disappointing results obtained with antisecretory agents, particularly in terms of a reduction in the lethality rate (Table 31), the questions arise whether they have not been used at an early enough stage and/or whether the pancreas becomes "immune" to the regulatory mechanisms for the intact organ in the state of acute pancreatitis.

10.4   Control of autodigestion and secondary inflammation

In keeping with prevailing concepts of the pathogenesis of acute pancreatitis, attempts have been made for more than two decades to interrupt the disease course, which is characterized by a high lethality rate, by administration of enzyme inhibitors. The studies cited in the literature – aside from individual reports about the use of elastase or phospholipase inhibitors – pertain to the protease inhibitor aprotinin (Trasylol®).

Table 31. Merits of pharmacological inhibition of pancreatic secretion in specific therapy of acute pancreatitis

Substance	Antisecretory mechanism	Efficacy in treatment of acute pancreatitis	Side effects	Comments
Anticholinergics (atropine)	Inhibition of hydro-kinetic and ecbolic pancreatic function; no effect on enzyme synthesis; inhibition of gastric acid secretion	No favorable effect demonstrable in doubleblind study of atropine [68]	Exacerbation of subileus and shock	Use inadvisable because of side effects
Carbonic anhydrase inhibitors (acetazolamide, Diamox®)	Inhibition of hydro-kinetic pancreatic function; no effect on enzyme secretion	Theoretically, not to be expected and not demonstrated in practice	Disturbances of electrolyte and acid-base metabolism; thickening of pancreatic secretions	Use disapproved [238]
Calcitonin	Inhibition of ecbolic pancreatic function; inhibition of gastric secretion	Improvement of clinical course but no drop in lethality rate [157, 359]	No side effects noted	Favorable effect not confirmed in another randomized study [509]
Glucagon	Inhibition of ecbolic and hydrokinetic pancreatic secretion and gastric secretion	No positive effect on course, no reduction of lethality [106, 256]	None observed	Usefulness unverified
Somatostatin	Inhibition of exocrine pancreatic secretion, gastric secretion, and of release of certain peptide hormones (e. g., gastrin, secretin, insulin, glucagon)	Animal study results contradictory, [274, 424] no controlled human studies available yet; preliminary observations optimistic [288, 462]	Insufficiently investigated; hyperosmolar coma reported [510]	Multicenter double-blind study now in progress [461]

10.4.1 Aprotinin

This protease inhibitor forms reversible equimolar complexes with trypsin, by which all zymogens of the pancreas, including prekallikrein, are activated [127], as well as with chymotrypsin, plasmin, and kallikrein, which − like trypsin − liberates kinins from kininogen (for review see Fritz et al. [135]). The residual proteolytic activity toward lower molecular weight peptides which remains demonstrable despite the binding of trypsin to α_2-macroglobulin can also be inhibited by aprotinin [33] (see Chapter 3).

The reasoning, based on these facts, that autodigestion and shock might be influenced by the administration of aprotinin (inhibition of kinin release) has been supported by experimental animal studies: a decrease of the lethality rate and reduction of shock effects have been observed in acute pancreatitis after aprotinin [176, 238, 450]. However, earliest possible use of the inhibitor is of critical importance for the therapeutic effect [230, 318, 450]. As Imrie and Mackenzie [230] were recently able to show in the dog, an experimentally induced biliary pancreatitis ended fatally in 100% of the cases when basic therapy alone was administered, whereas all the animals that received aprotinin also, 1 to 6 hours after induction of the pancreatitis, survived. Yet a mortality rate of 25% and 75%, respectively, was noted in animals that were treated after a delay of 9 and 12 hours.

In contrast to the preponderantly favorable animal study results, the clinical use of aprotinin (Trasylol®) remains controversial according to several reviews [103, 143, 158, 165, 238]. Remarkably, the debate between "opponents" and "proponents" of the drug has at times been emotionally colored. Apart from previous studies that were uncontrolled in many cases or conducted with insufficient doses, or both, the debate has mainly revolved around three double-blind studies on the use of aprotinin in acute pancreatitis [79, 229, 312, 458]. Although the lethality was significantly reduced by aprotinin (from 25% to 7.5%) according to Trapnell et al. [458], Imrie et al. [229] and the Multicentre Trial Group [79, 312] found both lethality and morbidity to be unaffected. Besides different selection criteria, the latent period that was allowed to elapse in the individual studies between the onset of the first symptoms and the beginning of treatment may be assumed to be primarily responsible for these divergent results. Thus, Trapnell et al. [458] limited their study to patients having their first attack of biliary or idiopathic pancreatitis, whereas the two other studies [79, 229, 312] also included alcoholic pancreatitis, for example, which usually runs a chronic relapsing course. Moreover, the Multicentre Trial Group [79, 312] admitted patients who had had acute attacks previously. With respect to the time lapse between onset of the first symptoms and the start of treatment, Trapnell et al. [458] made a distinction between administration after 24 hours and within the first 24 hours and found the mortality rate to be lower in the second group. This clinical trend is quite consistent with the experimental animal studies conducted by Imrie and Mackenzie [230]; (see above). In the clinical study preceding their experimental studies, on the other hand, Imrie et al. [229] began treatment within 48−60 hours after outbreak of the disease, whereas the Multicentre Trial Group [312] set a limit of 72 hours after the onset of the disease as the exclusion criterion. The high lethality rate in Trapnell et al. [458] placebo group that was criticized by some authors may have been attributable to the difference in patient selection and to the fact that the study period was less recent (1967 to 1972) than that in the other two studies.

Summing up our conclusions, we − in common with Back [25], Soergel [438], and DiMagno [99] − regard the data presented by Trapnell et al. [458] as valid evidence. In view of the contrary findings made in the two other studies, the disapproving attitude of other authors [158, 220, 268] toward aprotinin, the general uncertainty regarding the use of aprotinin, and the as yet unproved therapeutic alternatives, it will be necessary to carry out additional controlled studies in a precisely defined patient population, in whom the shortest possible time should be allowed to pass between the outbreak of the disease and the initiation of aprotinin therapy. This recommendation is supported by observations of the favorable effect of prophylactically administered aprotinin on postoperative pancreatitis [107, 199].

Attention should be called to the appearance of individual, extremely rare, anaphylactic reactions to aprotinin (31 out of 100,000 treated patients [177, 316]), occurring particularly after repeated use of the inhibitor. The duration of the treatment depends on the individual case. As a rule, treatment is useful only during the first few days. Continuation of the treatment for more than 5 days appears, for pathophysiological reasons, to offer little chance of success in most cases.

10.4.2   Other enzyme inhibitors

Besides the basic trypsin-kallikrein inhibitor aprotinin, the use of an elastase inhibitor and of epsilon-aminocaproic acid (EACA) and its derivatives, 4-aminomethylcyclohexanecarboxylic acid (AMCA) and p-aminomethylbenzoic acid (PAMBA), has been considered. These last inhibit plasmin and trypsin and reportedly increase the inhibitor pool of the plasma by this means. Animal study results are contradictory, and the clinical efficacy is disputed as shown in several reviews [51, 103, 143, 266]. Further studies are needed to arrive at a definite conclusion.

Owing to the pathophysiological significance of phospholipase A_2 in acute pancreatitis [343], the phospholipase A_2 inhibitor $CaNa_2EDTA$ was recently tentatively used in the treatment of acute pancreatitis [460]. As only 6 patients were treated, the optimism-inducing results should be evaluated with caution.

10.4.3   Indomethacin, acetylsalicylic acid, and prostaglandins

Whereas Lankisch [266] noted a life-prolonging effect of indomethacin in the experimental pancreatitis of the rat, Olazabal and Nascimento [351] observed an aggravation when they gave indomethacin or acetylsalicylic acid to rats. There have been no clinical studies with these two compounds or with protaglandins. Animal experimental data so far available on the effect of prostaglandin E_2 [270, 305] and prostaglandin I_2 [141] do not warrant their clinical use.

10.4.4   Antibiotics

The long-recommended prophylactic administration of antibiotics is controversial, at least in mild to moderately severe pancreatitis, beause the culture of resistant microorganisms may hamper antibiotic therapy when this becomes a necessity in addition to surgery, e.g., in the presence of abscesses [103, 225, 269]. In severe cases, notably in biliary reflux pancreatitis or when an abscess or sepsis is suspected, broad-spectrum antibiotics passing into the bile should be used specifically, in appropriately high doses and, if possible, on the basis of sensitivity tests, e.g., following bacteriological examination of drained secreta (see 10.6.3).

10.4.5   Therapeutic peritoneal lavage (peritoneal dialysis)

Besides diagnostic peritoneal lavage [311] (see 6.1.2.1), peritoneal dialysis is employed as "therapeutic peritoneal lavage" in acute pancreatitis. Technical details have been given by Stone and Fabian [443] and Ranson [369]. In this procedure, special attention has to be paid to the control of fluid balance (CVP!) and to pulmonary complications (see Chapter 11). It is the purpose of this treatment to remove from the abdominal cavity enzymes, kinins, and other toxic substances contained in the exudate and possibly also liquefied necrotized material or abscess contents. This prevents these substances from being absorbed by the peritoneum, which has a high absorptive capacity owing to its large surface area, and becoming systemically active. The course and complications of acute hemorrhagic-necrotizing pancreatitis can thus be benefited. This assumption rests on pathophysiological observations and experimental animal studies [28, 199, 490]. Clinical studies have produced encouraging results [369, 443] and several reviews have been published [103, 143, 156, 158, 266]. According to studies by Ranson [369], lethality in the early phase of the disease was significantly reduced by peritoneal lavage, and the clinical course was decisively ameliorated. This effect was attributed to action influencing early cardiovascular and pulmonary complications. The onset of late complications such as abscess formation and sepsis, however, was not prevented by peritoneal lavage, and the subsequent disease course was unaffected. The reduction in total lethality – insofar as this was at all possible in the individual groups being compared – was disappointingly small. By contrast, Stone and Fabian [443], who limited their study to patients with alcoholic pancreatitis, observed a marked reduction in overall lethality, particularly when the initially nondialyzed 17 out of 36 patients in the control group who were later subjected to peritoneal dialysis for ethical reasons, because of their clinically unfavorable course, were included in the comparison. Then only 8 of the total of 51 dialyzed patients died as compared with 6 of 19 patients in the control group. The divergent results might be due to the different selection criteria, particularly regarding etiology. Further controlled studies are needed to make a conclusive judgment. According to the data now on hand, the use of therapeutic peritoneal lavage seems justified as an adjunctive measure after weighing of the risk (e.g., infection, hemorrhage) in appropriate clinical situations (e.g., in shock) [158].

10.4.6   Improvement of pancreatic blood flow and microcirculation

Animal studies have shown that pancreatic blood flow and microcirculation are improved by the administration of low molecular weight dextrans, heparin, fibrinolytic therapy, sympathectomy, or ganglionic blockade. The clinical course and lethality rate are said to be favorably affected (see Lankisch [266] for review). Except for a prospective study with dextran 40, in which a positive trend emerged in the treatment of moderately severe but not of severe acute pancreatitis [39], controlled clinical studies on the effectiveness of these measures have not been conducted so far [103, 143, 158]. Their use cannot be recommended at this time for that reason. One should guard particularly against prophylactic administration of heparin and other antithrombotics in acute hemorrhagic-necrotizing pancreatitis, given the danger of bleeding complications (see 10.6.5).

10.5   Elimination of etiological factors

The recommendation that etiological factors of acute pancreatitis be eliminated as far as possible in order to influence the disease course is persuasive and compelling. That a drug capable of inducing acute pancreatitis should be withdrawn goes without saying (see Chapter 2). On the other hand, the presence of cholecystolithiasis should not ipso facto lead to cholecystectomy during the acute disease phase (see Chapter 11; see also Ranson [368]).

For biliary reflux pancreatitis provoked by concrements in the distal choledochus or the papillary region, *endoscopic papillotomy* (EPT) represents a recently introduced treatment modality carrying little risk. Results so far reported in the literature [393, 394, 463] and our own as yet unpublished observations [185] give grounds for unreserved endorsement of the earliest possible use of this procedure in *biliary reflux pancreatitis.*

Upon sonographic detection of cholelithiasis with congestion of the biliary tract the papilla is inspected with a side-viewing endoscope. The papilla usually has a balloon-like protrusion (Fig. 62, Plate XIII). Hereafter, the common bile duct is carefully filled with contrast medium in retrograde fashion and so visualized, after which a papillotomy is performed (Fig. 63, Plate XIII). If the stones do not (as in Fig. 64, Plate XIII) pass spontaneously, they should be extracted with the Dormia basket to provide for unimpeded efflux (Fig. 65).

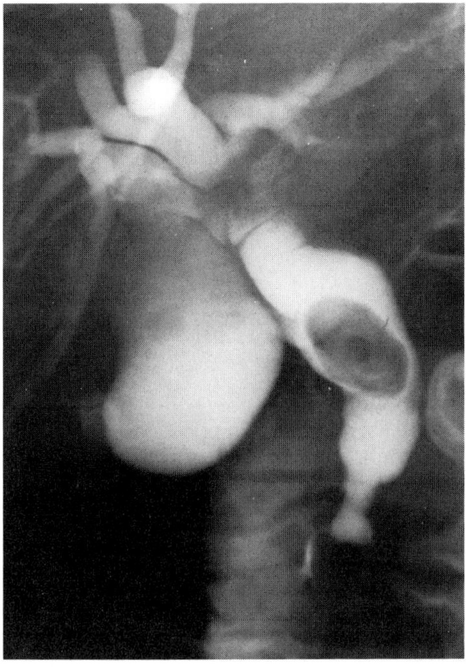

Fig. 65. Extraction of a choledochal concrement with Dormia basket.
(a) Cholecysto- and choledocholithiasis with congestion of bile ducts (endoscopic retrograde cholangiography prior to endoscopic papillotomy).

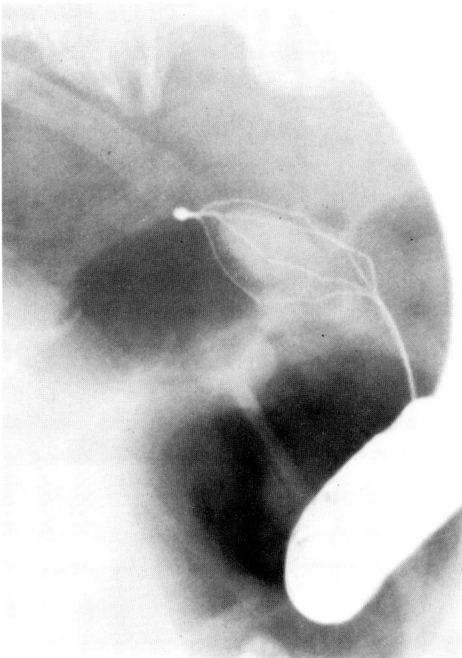

Fig. 65. Extraction of a choledochal concrement with Dormia basket.
(b) The choledochal stone that did not pass spontaneously after the endoscopic papillotomy is extracted with the Dormia basket (calculus in basket).

Cholecystectomy is desirable after abatement of the acute pancreatitis, not only in order to remove the risk (cholecystolithiasis) but also to prevent cholecystitis (due to ascending infection), which occurs more frequently after papillotomy. If complete drainage of the choledochal duct cannot be accomplished by EPT, the bile ducts have to be cleared surgically without delay (see Chapter 11). In acute pancreatitis not induced by biliary reflux, EPT is unlikely to be successful for pathogenetic reasons (see Chapter 4). It would, moreover, entail loss of papillary function and the gallbladder or, if cholecystectomy is not performed, an increased risk of cholecystitis.

10.6   Prevention and treatment of complications

Intensive surveillance of the patient makes it possible to prevent or at least detect at an early stage any complications that may arise. Basic recommendations are given at the beginning of this chapter.

10.6.1   Shock

This gravest of complications is brought about by volume deficiency as well as by the release of kinins. Basic therapy includes the adequate administration of fluid, electrolytes, and albumin while the CVP is being monitored and, if necessary, of blood. Dextran

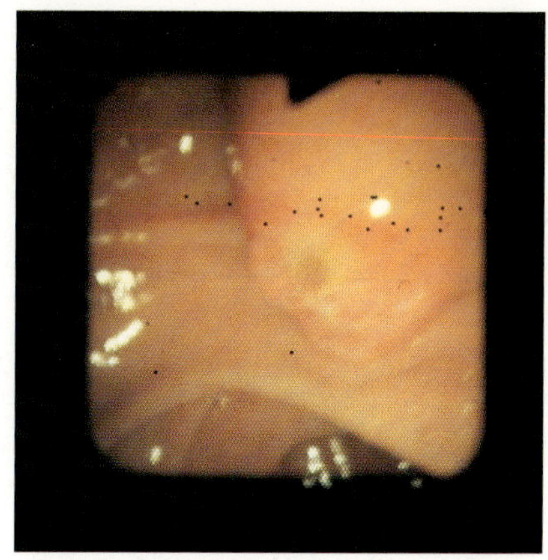

Fig. 62. Ballooning papilla with necrotic porus papillae in a cholecystectomized female patient, age 62, with recurrent stones in choledochus, obstructive jaundice, cholangitis, and pancreatitis.

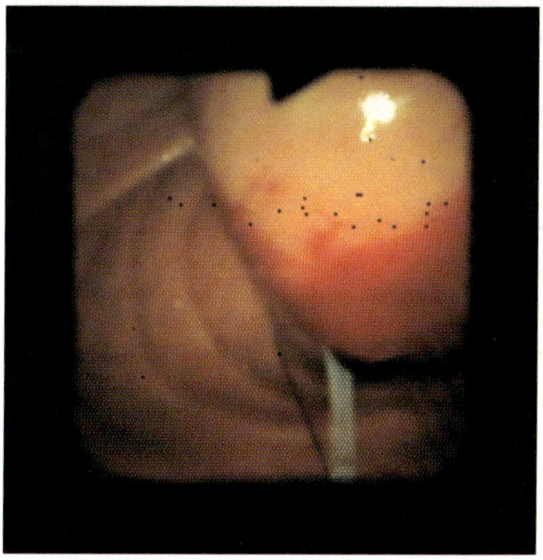

Fig. 63. Papillotom is inserted into common bile duct, and stretched (same patient as in Fig. 62).

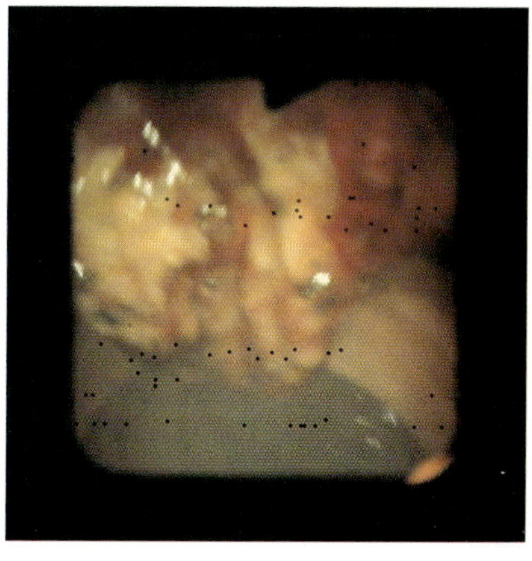

Fig. 64. Spontaneous "delivery" of stone (same patient as in Fig. 63); after papillotomy there was rapid clinical improvement with normalization of serum lipase level and remission of leukocytosis.

Plate XIII

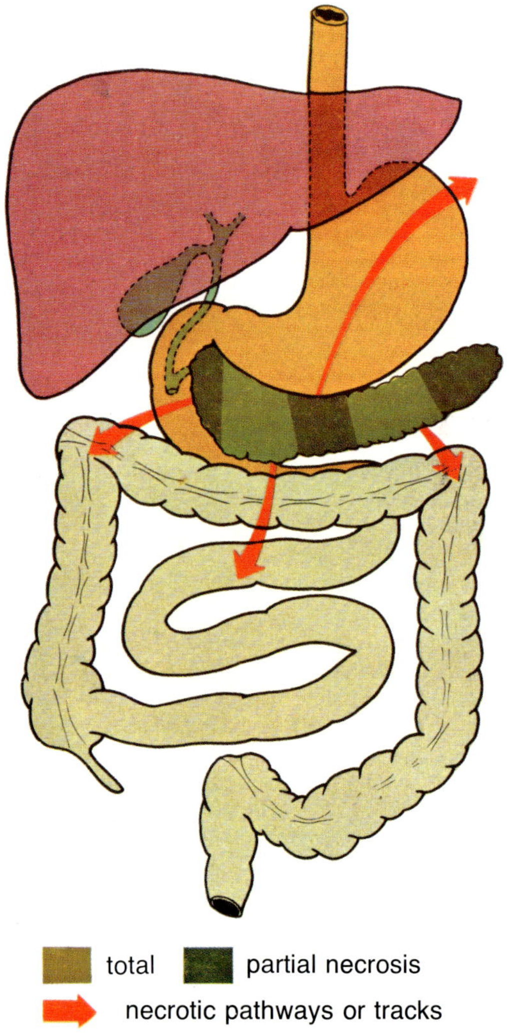

Fig. 66. Extension of parenchymal necrosis and peripancreatic necrosis to so-called necrotic pathways. (From M. Neher, G. Mangold, K. Rückert, and F. Kümmerle: Pankreaschirurgie, Med. Klin. 75: 613, 1980.)

Plate XIV

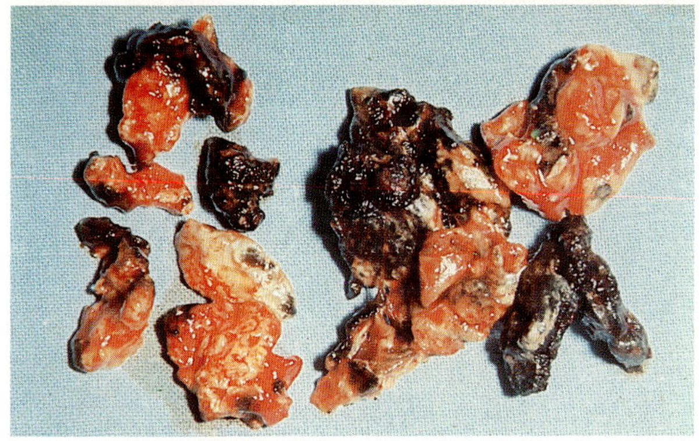

Fig. 67. Multiple partial ectomies of necrotized pancreatic tissue.

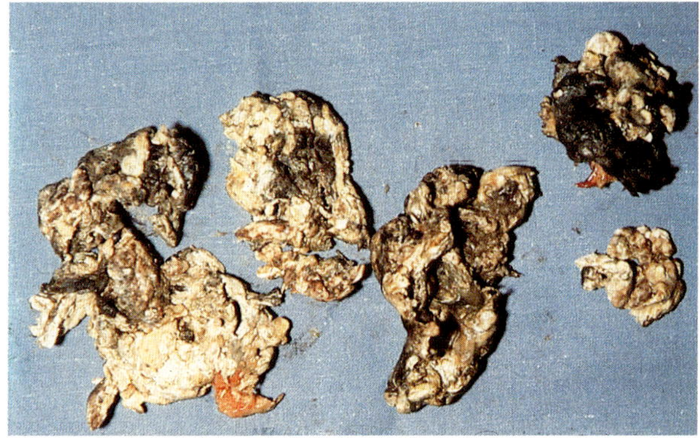

Fig. 68. Multiple pancreatic sequestra after sequestrectomy with clearly visible "saponification".

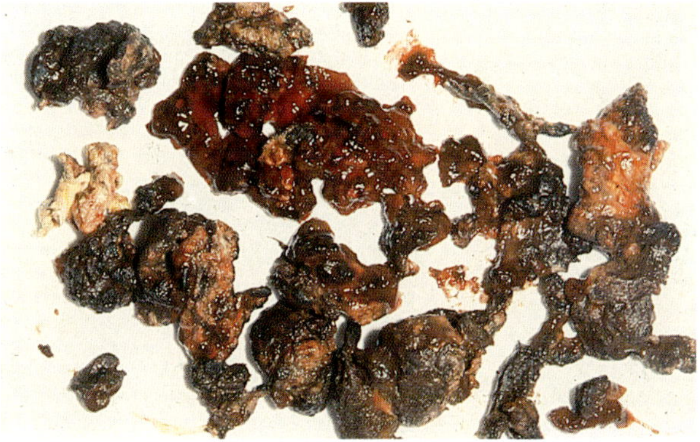

Fig. 69. Mixed portions of necrotized pancreas with pancreatic sequestra.

Plate XV

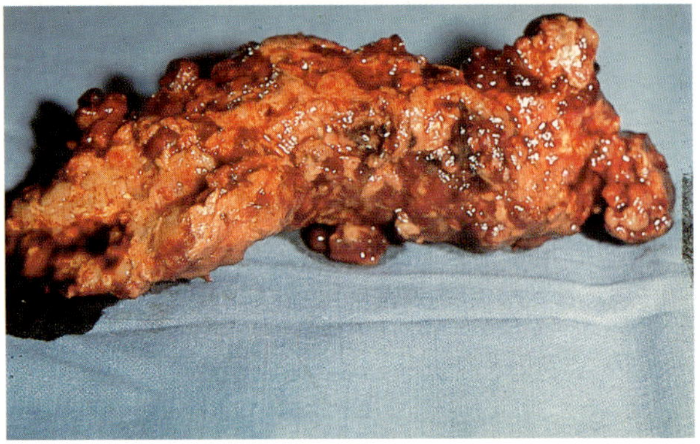

Fig. 70. Pancreatic resection: so-called subtotal resection in hemorrhagic-necrotizing pancreatitis.

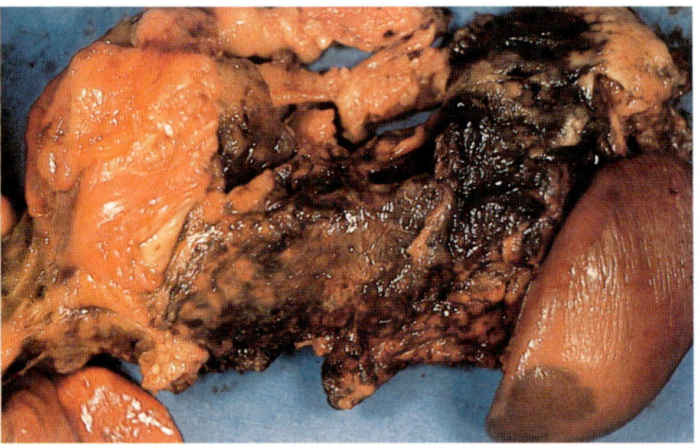

Fig. 71. Pancreatic resection in presence of necrosis in isthmic, body, and tail regions with splenectomy.

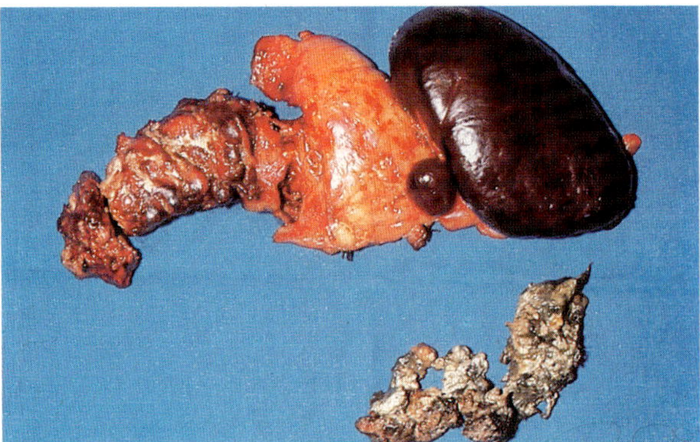

Fig. 72. Pancreatic resection of isthmus, corpus, and tail with removal of a left-sided necrotic pathway and splenectomy.

Plate XVI

solutions should be given only after weighing of the risks (hemorrhage) considering their antithrombotic effect [169]. As Balldin and Ohlsson [32] showed in animal studies, aprotinin may exert an additional advantageous effect in shock by virtue of its action on the kallikrein-kinin system. Peritoneal lavage, too, eliminates enzymes, kinins, and other toxic substances from the body. If necessary, dopamine and dobutamine may be given as well [268]. In common with Goebell and Dürr [158], we disapprove of the administration of corticosteroids, since these may have a deleterious effect on the course of acute pancreatitis (see Chapter 2).

10.6.2 Renal and pulmonary insufficiency

The onset of renal insufficiency calls for institution of dialysis therapy. This should begin as early as possible, and underlying causes should be eliminated whenever possible (e.g., surgical intervention in septicemic renal failure). In respiratory insufficiency, assisted or controlled ventilation under positive end-expiratory pressure (PEEP) should be initiated early in keeping with the blood gas analysis. Mechanical disorders such as pleural effusions have to be removed by puncture, and the punctate must be analyzed diagnostically (protein, enzyme concentrations, microbiological study; also cytology for differential diagnosis; see Chapter 3).

A beneficial effect of aprotinin in shock lung has been reported by Boumghar and Cavin [54].

10.6.3 Local complications and sepsis

When a secondary bacterial infection is discovered or suspected, specific antibiotic therapy should be instituted (see 10.4.4) and, if need be, timely surgical intervention (e.g., in case of abscess formation, infected pseudocysts). Regular sonographic follow-up examinations and, if available, computed tomography are indicated.

Since heparin is primarily contraindicated in acute hemorrhagic-necrotizing pancreatitis, it must not be routinely administered in the presence of sepsis (danger of consumption coagulopathy) but should be used only after precise coagulation tests have been ascertained and the risks (also at lower doses) weighed (see 10.6.5).

In the presence of bland pseudocysts intervention may be delayed unless signs of local displacement require immediate action. Pseudocysts developing in the course of acute pancreatitis regress in about 25% of cases; they become chronic in 50% and lead to complications in another 25% (see Hollender and Marrie [209] and Chapters 8 and 11).

Hollender [199] recommends aprotinin–also for local use–in the treatment of fistulas (see Chapter 8). According to our own observations in individual cases, somatostatin, too, has a beneficial effect.

10.6.4 Diabetes mellitus

Hyperglycemia and, at times, hypoglycemia can develop in acute pancreatitis. Reference has been made above to the need for continuous monitoring of the serum glucose level. Diabetes mellitus has to be treated with insulin. One should make certain that small doses of the easily controllable regular insulin (unmodified insulin) are infused intravenously (Perfusor!) since counterregulation may no longer be operative (glucagon deficiency) in the presence of advanced organ destruction. It will then be necessary to inject glucagon. Concomitant glucose infusions, together with glucose substitutes (fructose, xylitol), are part of the basic management program. In renal failure, the insulin dose should be reduced since there is a reduced insulin clearance.

10.6.5   Coagulation defects

Hypo- as well as hypercoagulopathies may occur in the course of an acute pancreatitis [238]. Besides consumption coagulopathy in sepsis and thrombotic complications, disseminated intravascular coagulation presents therapeutic problems [508]. Since acute hemorrhagic-necrotizing pancreatitis per se (see Chapter 4) is a contraindication for anticoagulant therapy, heparin may be given only–even in low doses–after the (doubtful) benefits have been carefully weighed against the risks. The coagulation tests should be checked regularly (also, among other things, for deficiency of antithrombin III, for example) and, if necessary, supplementation of specific individual factors (e.g., antithrombin III), and possibly the use of enzyme inhibitors as an alternative to low-dose heparin therapy, should be considered [418].

10.7   Concluding remarks

Conservative therapy suffices in the clinically mild "edematous" pancreatitis ("severity grade" I). In the presence of cholecystolithiasis without concomitant choledocholithiasis and without congestion of the bile ducts, cholecystectomy may be delayed until the interval. The decision whether and when to operate is difficult in the case of acute hemorrhagic-necrotizing pancreatitis severity grades II and III (see Chapters 4 and 5). The onset of complications e.g., abscesses, makes the decision easier. The criteria for surgical intervention are discussed in Chapter 11.

Chapter 11 – Surgical Therapy

11.1 Indications for surgery

Surgical therapy of acute pancreatitis is a problem that will always be current. Nordmann's report from the year 1938 in which he summarized his unfavorable experience with the surgically oriented treatment of acute pancreatitis by concluding that he should forgo laparotomy and surgical intervention has been a milestone in the history of surgery in pancreatitis.

The subsequently practiced "active internistic therapy" of acute pancreatitis has today reached its highest standard in following an interdisciplinary intensive care approach utilizing tremendously improved diagnostic methods for developmental control. However, the exclusive reliance on internistic, conservative intensive care is of limited usefulness in the specifically pancreatitic autodigestive disease and the constant danger of progressive or recurrent necrosis it presents [330].

For these reasons a further improvement of treatment results cannot be expected without interruption of the local inflammatory process in the organ, and patients with progressive or newly arising, and consequently fatal, sequential complications are forever under the threat of an unfavorable prognosis [330].

In the light of these fundamental considerations regarding indications for surgery, and taking due note of the clinical experience that severe necrotic forms of pancreatitis are bound to end fatally despite the use of all resources of intensive medical care, a carefully planned surgical therapy may and should be pursued–as a complementary measure, not a competing alternative–under the following conditions provided certain criteria are satisfied:

(1) when the diagnosis is uncertain;
(2) when biliary pancreatitis has been established;
(3) in pancreatitis-induced local or referred, frequently septic, complications due to infected necrotic tissue and necrotic pathways;
(4) as a general rule, when the general condition worsens or fails to improve despite optimal conservative treatment.

The *goal* of a surgical procedure always is the elimination of necrotic tissue segments at the optimal time. Residual necroses are irreversible processes predisposing to persistence which develop and expand from the retro-peritoneal pancreatic compartment in the form of necrotic pathways (Fig. 66, Plate XIV).

The *tactics* and *techniques* of the operation must be based, aside from the local findings, on the disease course and developmental trend, and in addition to eliminating an existing complication, the operation should also have a causal-pathogenetic orientation regarding sonography and CT.

The question whether to reoperate or repeat laparotomy must be determined by the clinical symptomatology, vital parameters being taken into consideration. All carefully evaluated clinical and surgical observations attest to the possibility of improving the chances for survival in these most severe forms of pancreatitis if the criteria outlined above are heeded. Regardless of the local process, surgical intervention is a vital necessity whenever a finding of acute abdomen–due to peritonitis and hemorrhage–is made that requires clarification.

11.2 Specific surgical therapy

The evolutive pathogenesis and the clinical polymorphism of acute pancreatitis should thus be matched by a highly differentiated surgical approach and a discriminating choice of cases suitable for surgery.

The conservative medical treatment always indicated at the outset should conform to the guidelines given in the preceding chapter.

The exception is the case in which the diagnosis is doubtful or uncertain. This means that exploratory-diagnostic laparotomy is necessary in all situations of acute or sub-acute abdomen the type and etiology of which cannot be definitely established. If the laparotomy reveals pancreatitis, the actions to be taken from then on depend on the nature of the pathological changes encountered, their topography, and their extra-pancreatic spread. We shall come back to this point later on.

Under the positive influence of intense therapeutic measures, notably the control of pancreatitis-induced life-threatening states of shock, the acute pancreatitis can assume or pass through at different times several degrees of severity that patients could not have survived in the past. They will dictate the decision whether or not to operate. The manifold courses and degrees of severity of acute pancreatitis are divided into three grades of severity according to the efficacy of conservative medical treatment (Table 32).

The first grade continues, as a general rule, to be treated conservatively. Pancreatitis cases of the third grade of severity, on the other hand, nearly all end fatally, even after surgical therapy. Thus, surgical therapy may be worth considering mainly in variants of the second grade of severity (see below for specific operative measures).

Gall suggests that an endoscopic radiogram be taken of the duct of Wirsung immediately before the operation (private communication). Pancreatography provides information on possible lesions in the pancreatic duct, and on this basis the operative tactics to be employed can be determined at the very beginning of the operation [23, 56, 57, 114, 205, 214, 216, 257, 259, 416, 417].

Table 32. Classification of acute pancreatitis by morphological, clinical, and biological criteria (degrees of severity according to Hollender and Kümmerle, 209, 258).

Grade 1: Edematous pancreatitis

Clinical:
Epigastric pain +
Vomiting (±)

Epigastric tenderness (+)
Slight guarding (+)
No jaundice
BP >120
Pulse ~ 100/min

Good response to conservative
therapy

Laboratory parameters:
No serious abnormalities in:
– Blood sugar
– Serum calcium
– BUN and creatinine
– Hematocrit
Serum amylase ↑
Urine amylase ↑
Serum lipase ↑
Progressive normalization of pancreatic
enzymes under conservative therapy

Grade 2: Limited pancreatic necroses

Clinical: *Laboratory parameters:*
Epigastric pain + +   Leukocytosis (>15,000/μl)
Vomiting +, tachypnea   Hematocrit $\downarrow\downarrow$
Diffuse abdominal pain,   BUN $\uparrow$, creatinine $\uparrow$
most severe   Blood sugar ($\uparrow$) (<150 mg/dl)
in epigastrium (guarding +,   Serum calcium $\downarrow$ (2 mmol/l)
meteorism +, subileus +,   Serum amylase $\uparrow\uparrow$
resistance in upper abdomen [+])   Serum lipase $\uparrow\uparrow$
Subicterus to icterus, progressive   Puncture of abdomen: brownish,
BP <100   enzymerich fluid
Pulse >120/min   (Peritoneal lavage,
Temperature ~ 38° C   laparoscopy)

High fluid requirement of more than 3 l/24 h to keep central venous pressure constant and maintain urine excretion.
Little or no response to conservative treatment!

Grade 3: Diffuse necrotizing pancreatitis (with/without extrapancreatic exudation, pleural effusion, retrocolic pathways of necrosis)

Clinical: *Laboratory parameters:*
As in grade 2:   Leukocytosis   >20,000/μl
Signs of shock + +/CVP!!   Blood sugar   >150 mg/dl
Increasing oliguria + +   Serum calcium   <2 mmol/l
                                                   Metabolic acidosis
Respiratory insufficiency + +   Hypoxia
Encephalopathy +   Hypocapnia
Gastrointestinal hemorrhage (+)   Transaminases $\uparrow$
Hematocrit (decrease)   Creatinine/BUN $\uparrow\uparrow$
                                                   Serum amylase $\varnothing/\uparrow\uparrow$
BP <80/CVP!   Serum lipase $\varnothing/\uparrow\uparrow$
Pulse >140/min   Lethal factors!
Temperature 38–39° C   (See Ranson's prognostic index)
Notably high fluid demand

Progressive exacerbation despite conservative intensive treatment!

11.2.1   Timing of operation

The choice of the right or most advantageous time for surgery is difficult and problematical.

This decision can never be arrived at on theoretical grounds.

Experience has shown, however, that it would be wrong to maintain that the operation has to be carried out within the first 24 hours or after 24 hours or between the 1st and 3rd days or between the 3rd and 6th days. Optimal timing of the surgical intervention is of critical importance. By the same token, unduly elaborate and superfluous measures must be avoided. On the other hand, no operation should be forced, particularly if the operative site makes an immediate operation appear inappropriate, or if this can no longer be realized.

In actual practice, the clinical and specifically the abdominal response to conservative treatment will serve as a guide.

Continuously progressive worsening of the general condition or a new exacerbation after transient improvement, the development of a so-called enzymatic pancreatic encephalopathy or respiratory insufficiency, aggravation of jaundice or subicterus, a new or increasing pleural effusion, epigastric guarding, increasing oliguria or threatening renal failure with marked increases in the blood levels of urea nitrogen and creatinine, the onset of metabolic acidosis, persistent hypocalcemia, and the onset of leukocytosis despite optimal intensive therapy–all these are signs which, appearing either singly or in combination, argue in favor of the need for surgery in conjunction with close, complex, and differential surveillance using sonography and, possibly, computed tomography (see Chapter 6). Here again, the timing is of crucial diagnostic and therapeutic significance [192, 193, 194, 195, 196].

11.2.2   Operative modalities

Two principal considerations and actions are involved in any procedure that is undertaken in the course of an acute pancreatitis:

11.2.2.1   Biliary tract operations

11.2.2.1.1   Cholecystectomy
If cholecystolithiasis without choledochal lithiasis and without obstruction of the biliary tract has been established, it is advisable to wait a few days while continuing strict clinical and sonographic monitoring. After 1 week at the latest the cholecystectomy should then be performed. In an unfavorable case, corrective action by cholecystectomy and complete clearance of the bile ducts have to be effected rapidly with intraoperative cholangiography and choledochoscopy.

11.2.2.1.2   Choledochal exploration
In *choledocholithiasis,* an attempt is first made to remove the concrements endoscopically. One must be certain, however, that all stones are removed during this first treatment. If this is not accomplished, operative removal of the stones or correction of the obstruction is imperative. If a stone-free bile duct system can be obtained by endoscopic papillary and bile duct exploration, the operation may be delayed.

Whether an operation is indicated will then depend on the further course as related to the pancreatitic findings.

11.2.2.2   Operation on the pancreas: Inspection and exploration

The procedure depends on the *local findings.* Broad opening of the pancreatic compartment and complete exposure of the pancreas permit precise evaluation of the organ's condition. An extensive so-called Kocher maneuver with broad transection of the gastrocolic ligament and detachment of the pancreatic tail with the spleen make possible a thorough examination of the entire organ.

Before one or the other approach is decided upon, the pancreatic capsule has to be broadly incised in longitudinal direction and the pancreas carefully examined. Only thus is it possible to determine exactly that a macroscopically normal pancreas is concealed under an edematously infiltrated capsule, or that the lesions are for the most part in peripancreatic locations or that, in the opposite case, hemorrhagic-necrotic foci exist beneath a pancreatic capsule showing only slight edematous changes [197, 198, 199, 200, 201, 202].

For the pancreas itself, a whole series of distinct operative procedures may be applicable.

11.2.3 Operative procedures in acute pancreatitis: Drainage and irrigation

As a *minimal local operation, peripancreatic and intraperitoneal drainage* with therapeutic *irrigation* may be considered. In this procedure several perforated drains are inserted in the pancreatic compartment to permit adequate, reliable irrigation. Within 24 hours 10–12 liters of a 0.9% saline solution or, preferably, a peritoneal dialysate of the following composition are perfused:

NaCl, 5.6 g;
sodium lactate, 5.09 g;
$CaCl_2$, 0.52 g;
$MgCl_2$, 0.15 g;
glucose, 15 g;
twice-distilled water to make 1000 ml
(osmolarity, 360 mosmol/l).

With the use of a potassium-free lavage fluid, supplemental K^+ has to be administered intravenously.

The lavage fluid perfuses large-caliber drains (minimum inside diameter, 1.5 cm) so that necrotic debris may be aspirated or washed out. The drains are placed alongside the pancreas, in the right-sided and left-sided coloparietal spaces, and in the Douglas pouch.

Maroske, Thon, and Röher [304] recently reported on their experience with therapeutic peritoneal lavage in terms of its effect on the need for surgery and drew the following conclusions:

1. If the initial therapeutic peritoneal lavage is successful, demarcation of necrotic and abscessed areas may be awaited. This creates more favorable conditions for definitive surgery; an immediate, stressful laparotomy in the acute initial phase of this serious disease is then avoided in the clinical presence of diffuse peritonitis.

2. Regular bacteriological examinations of the peritoneal exudate (dialysate), catheter urine, and possibly blood cultures are a requirement if a specific antibiotic therapy is to be instituted.

Removal of necrotized tissue
This takes the form of an elective removal by digitoclasia or scalpel, defined areas of necrosis being severed from the healthy parenchyma. This can be done most advantageously if the necrotic areas are still "dry" (Fig. 67, Plate XV).

Sequestrectomies
They are performed in the case of advanced, "moist" necrosis in the stage of liquefaction. Variously sized fragments of dead pancreas with a purulent or infected fluid having become detached from the pancreas are ablated (depending on the particular case) (Fig. 68, Plate XV). It may be necessary to remove a completely infarcted pancreas that no longer has any vascular connections (Fig. 69, Plate XV).

Segmental resections
Necrotized pancreatic segments of varying size can be resected by digitoclasia or, depending on the nature and stage of the pancreatitic process, by the "normal" procedure. The resections are done from left to right, or from the tail toward the head of the pancreas. They are ended at the point where healthy pancreatic tissue is discernible (Fig. 70, Plate XVI).

Segmental resections and removal of necrotized tissue may be combined, the resection being extended as far as the superior mesenteric vein and necrotized tissue being removed in the head region (Fig. 67).

Total gastroduodenopancreatectomy
In view of the unforeseeable development of certain variants of necrotizing pancreatitis of the greatest severity, involving necrotic alterations of the entire pancreas, and because of the risk of allowing foci of necrosis to remain and spread, thus sustaining the disease and causing it to progress, several authors removed the entire pancreas with the duodenum and two-thirds of the stomach [5, 6, 7]. This radical operation is said to have been successful in otherwise hopeless cases. However, this is a lengthy, difficult, bloodlosing operation that ought to be performed only by an experienced and practiced surgical team.

11.2.4 Laparostomy: "open abdomen"

This treatment of the laparotomy wound has been recommended for some time now by several pancreatic surgery centers for the most severe forms of intraperitoneal infection as the newest special therapeutic method for acute necrotizing pancreatitis with intraperitoneal complications, notably peritonitis.

It consists in leaving the abdomen wide open after the laparotomy and in covering the small bowel loops only with the greater omentum or, if this is not possible, with a film. This allows easy outflow of exudates and transudates.

At the same time repeated, extensive peritoneal cleaning with manual removal of necrotic debris and accumulations of pus – regardless of their localization – including pancreatic and peripancreatic necrotic tissue and abscesses can be accomplished with ease.

The advantage of such an open laparotomy treatment, permitting optimal cleaning of the abdominal cavity, is evident. The cleaning operation is performed as often as necessary, generally three to five times at intervals of 24–48 hours, depending finally on the individual findings.

Such a laparostomy is indicated for the most part with repeat intervention in the presence of large masses of necrotized tissue or multiple abscesses. In the most severe cases with disseminated foci of necrosis it may also be done at the first laparotomy.

11.2.5   Adjunctive procedures: Biliary tract operations

Independently of measures to be taken locally on the pancreas, it is advisable to remove the gallbladder as well (insofar as this is technically feasible) and to effect drainage of the choledochus by means of a T-drain according to Kehr. Such a discharge by outward diversion of the bile is advantageous also in the absence of lithiasis. If manipulations and measures on the common bile duct are too difficult because of excessive edema in the hepatoduodenal ligament, the operation will have to be limited to simple cholecystectomy or, in problem cases to cholecystotomy (see 11.2.3).

Choledochal stones must definitely be removed and eliminated by choledochotomy. If a stone is lodged in the ampulla of Vater that can neither be removed endoscopically nor moved into the duodenum by choledochotomy, transduodenal sphincterotomy is indicated–a most unusual case. It should be borne in mind that, if at all possible, any enterotomy ought to be avoided or circumvented in a situation of acute pancreatitis.

Some authors refrain from any action on the biliary tract unless lithiasis is ascertainable with absolute certainty (Kümmerle).

11.2.6   Adjunctive local procedures on the pancreas

Any operation on the pancreas (removal of necrotized tissue, exeresis, sequestrectomy) should be supplemented by broad lavage and drainage of the pancreatic compartment. Subcostally to the left, a wide-diameter-drain is inserted into the bursa parallel to the body of the pancreas, and another is placed in the right hypochondrium for discharge from the head of the pancreas. A third drain is used for the medial portion of the pancreas (cf. Fig. 71, Plate XVI). "Sump drainage".

Pancreatic fistulas often develop after the removal of necrotic tissue. It is important therefore to apply a separate through-drain for each drainage zone. Inflowing and outflowing drainage fluids are carefully measured so that electrolyte and fluid losses may be precisely checked.

11.2.7   Adjunctive measures in extrapancreatic necrosis

Areas of pancreatic necrosis must by all means be tracked down and eliminated also outside the pancreas, behind the ascending and descending colon, along the radix mesenterii, and as far as the pelvic floor (Figs. 67–69). For this purpose wide-lumen drains are introduced into the right and left parietocolic spaces so that their openings will be located in the posterior external portion of the hypochondrium or in the flanks.

In rare cases the transverse colon may exhibit sites of partial necrosis due to enzymatic digestion; a colon segment with such alterations has to be resected. The right and left colon are separately passed through the abdominal wall and infolded as a stoma.

11.3   Operative strategy

The specific surgical treatment should be based on four empirical guiding principles and fundamental concepts that can be derived from what has been said above:
1. Overly extensive and aggressive measures should be avoided.
2. The development of the hemorrhagic-necrotic changes in particular and the resultant appearance of complications should be monitored by means of ultrasonography and computed tomography in such a manner that surgical intervention can be undertaken immediately under optimal conditions, hence at the optimal time.
3. The prerequisite is exact, optimal infusion therapy.
4. Since the direction and timing of the disease course are unforeseeable, one has to be in readiness for one or more repeat operations at all times. Everyone involved in intensive treatment is bound to have learned that reintervention may be unavoidable and, indeed, imperative.

The four major variants of acute pancreatitis will be discussed below on the basis of these principles:

11.3.1   Acute pancreatitis of biliary origin

In these cases the logical therapeutic course to follow is removal of the obstruction impeding the flow of bile and pancreatic secretions.

Once a choledocholithiasis with obstruction has been established, the patient is first of all referred and entrusted to the care of an endoscopist experienced in papillotomy. After a careful examination and confirmation of the indication, endoscopic papillotomy with removal of the calculi and drainage of bile ducts and, in exceptional cases, the pancreatic duct has to be performed (see Chapter 10).

If this procedure is not successful, surgical intervention, viz., cholecystectomy, clearing of the bile ducts, and instrumental exploration of the choledochus, cannot be avoided. Additionally, choledochoscopy is important in the presence of impacted stones, which may be removed under choledochoscopic control. Thereafter, a T-drain is inserted for outward diversion of the bile. Only if the sphincter of Oddi cannot be unblocked by this canalicular route is it necessary to perform a transduodenal sphincterotomy. However, this is possible only in the absence of a marked inflammatory change and infiltration of the duodenal wall.

The following adjunctive measures are taken considering other local findings and the topography of the pancreatic necrosis:

Direct removal of areas of necrosis by caudal, corporeal-caudal pancreatectomy or removal of necrotized tissue. If the necrosis is "dry", however, the removal is not always easy to accomplish. Yet on the very first days the necrotized tissues are not yet "moist" and the sequestrum is clearly delineated from the normal parenchyma (Fig. 72, Plate XVI).

Peripancreatic drainage and irrigation.

If surgery on the pancreas was not yet necessary or indicated at the time of the first intervention, the patient should undergo regular sonographic and computed tomography examinations for follow-up observation. The findings then made may indicate the need for excision of necrotized areas or sequestrectomy.

11.3.2 Alcoholic pancreatitis

This presents different problems, if only because of the undetermined pathogenesis. Therefore, opinions about the nature and scope of the surgery to be performed still vary. The disease course is the determining factor. If the patient has a history of repeated subacute episodes of pancreatitis, no operation should be performed, and the same applies if the disease is of moderate severity clinically and in terms of laboratory values. However, in the event the patient's general condition worsens in spite of optimal conservative, intensive treatment and both sonography and computed tomography disclose increased pancreatic necrosis, caudal, corporeal or isthmic-corporeal-caudal exeresis is in order.

It is necessary to proceed with an early operation only in the presence of an extremely severe, fulminant necrotic pancreatitis. This is intervention as a last resort which, in the hands of an experienced surgeon, may not infrequently save the patient's life contrary to expectations [205, 206, 207, 208].

11.3.3 Postoperative pancreatitis

This form of inflammation has the special characteristic of developing rapidly. The majority of cases involve massive inflammatory changes. A combination of lipoproteolytic necrosis, extravasation of blood with threatening autodigestion of neighboring organs, particularly of the retropancreatic choledochus, of vessels close to the pancreas, and the duodenal region predominates. In cases of this severity any medical treatment is doomed to failure. Immediate surgical intervention, in the form of subtotal pancreatectomy from left to right, is an ineluctable necessity under these conditions provided a healthy pancreatic zone still exists in the duodenal region. Otherwise, duodenectomy with resection of the pancreatic head is the only possibility remaining. The prognosis is unfavorable from the start. Simple excision of the focus or foci of necrosis is not enough because the necrotizing process spreads to healthy tissues [203].

11.3.4 Posttraumatic pancreatitis

The specific operative procedure to be followed in cases of pancreatic involvement and suspected posttraumatic pancreatitis following blunt abdominal trauma does not lend itself to generalization. Essentially, posttraumatic pancreatitis requires the same approach—always depending on the individual organ findings—as other forms of pancreatitis. In the presence of early changes with no discernible ongoing autodigestive inflammation, the operative care will be based on the nature and location of the injury. As a rule, partial resection proves more effective, being more reliable in terms of the final outcome, than attempts to retain the organ intact. Treatment of pancreatic duct ruptures and deeper parenchymal ruptures by resection purposely avoids any attempt at reanastomosis of the pancreatic duct with a view to saving the organ. This approach also rests on the experience that in the absence of prior damage to the pancreas even substantial losses of parenchyma are tolerated without any serious excretory or incretory insufficiency. Any attempt at duct suture to retain the organ, on the other hand, may lead to numerous complications.

In every case of posttraumatic pancreatitis or posttraumatic pancreatic injury surgical exploration and care must always be followed by extensive drainage of the pancreatic compartment. As in diffuse septic peritonitis, through-drainage in particular offers special advantages since it promotes the removal of residual or newly formed necrotic products and also prevents possible fistula formation or drain retention (see Chapter 10, Conservative Therapy; Peritoneal lavage).

In the context of the release of proteases and the incubation of blood with proteases, the therapeutic principle of prophylactic or adjunctive protease inhibitor treatment in such severe problem cases is a well-established concept. Inhibitor therapy is justified if all therapeutic possibilities are to be exhausted, even if its effectiveness is not as yet satisfactorily demonstrable by clinical methods [190, 218, 336].

11.3.5 Idiopathic pancreatitis

The decision whether to operate is most difficult to make in patients with this form of pancreatitis. It will have to depend on the clinical condition and course with special reference to sonographic and computed tomography data. The operation may be exeresis as far as the radix mesenterii, with or without removal of necrotized tissues at the head or layer by layer.

11.4 Postoperative nutrition: Hyperalimentation

Patients with pancreatitis have to be assured of an adequate caloric intake, which should slowly increase to 60 calories/kg of body weight, or to about 4000–5000 calories in 24 hours (see Chapter 10.2.3).

Feeding is done parenterally at first. A sufficient caloric supply is an essential part of the treatment and should never be underestimated. In the first few days lipid supplementation should be kept low; starting with the 5th or 6th day, lipid administration may be slowly increased. As soon as the acute symptoms subside and ileus or subileus has ceased, a gradual transition to enteral nutrition is advisable. This can be done in two ways:

A double-lumen indwelling nasogastric tube is inserted via the pylorus into the first jejunal loop (Fig. 73).

Alternatively, the feeding tube may be inserted through a jejunostomy, preferably on the occasion of a laparotomy that needs to be done in any event.

Except in unusual cases, of course, laparotomy may not be performed for the sole purpose of providing such an alimentary jejunostomy.

The technique described by Delany involves antimesenteric insertion of an opaque nasogastric tube 91 cm long and 8 mm in diameter into the jejunal wall of the second loop and applying it in the form of a Witzel fistula. The tube is then aborally advanced into the lumen for another 30 cm, and when its position has been carefully checked by x-ray, the abdominal wall is punctured as for a Redon drain and the tube, in close contact with the wall, is then passed to the outside. The skin aperture is protected and cared for as with the use of a venous catheter.

If adequate caloric intake cannot be assured by this means in a nonlaparotomized patient, parenteral alimentation via a subclavian catheter is indispensable.

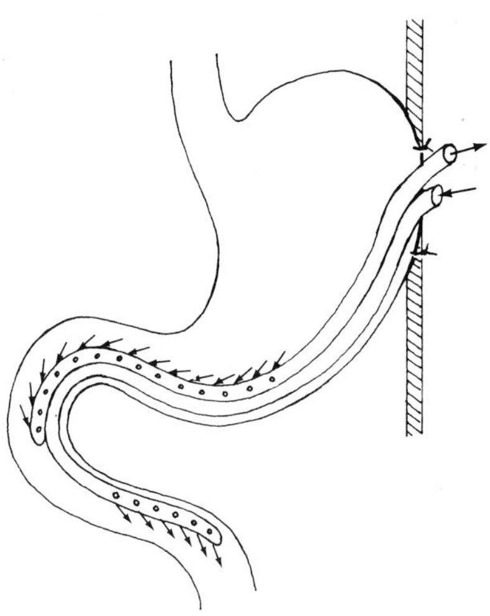

Fig. 73. Transgastric transduodenojejunal double-lumen suction and feeding tube.

As a general rule, however, enteral and, specifically, intrajejunal alimentation affords considerable advantages over parenteral alimentation since there is less risk of mechanical, metabolic, and especially septic complications than with parenteral feeding. Moreover, exclusively parenteral alimentation may entail side effects, to which far too little attention has been paid in the past. It is imperative to maintain digestive function through nutrient substrates in the intestine so that the hormone-stimulating trophic effect on the gastrointestinal mucosa may not be suspended for too long a time. Enteral nutrition is also far less costly [184].

The formerly shown reluctance to employ catheter jejunostomy is mainly attributable to the fact that both optimal nutrient compositions and desirable catheter materials for the jejunostomy have become available only now.

A not inconsequential advantage of this type of postoperative alimentation is the protection it affords against any serious patient discomfort. In contrast to nasogastric feeding (Table 33) intrajejunal tube alimentation is associated with virtually no complications due to vomiting and aspiration. Heberer was the first who recently published a convincing account of his experience with this thechnique in the German-language literature [206, 210, 211, 212, 213].

Table 33. Contraindications to nasogastric tube feeding in complications of pancreatitis

1. Suspected ileus (intestinal atony), persistent vomiting
2. Peptic esophagitis
3. Mechanical and functional side effects, local tube complications (erosion, ulcer, hermorrhage)

Note: The optimal positioning of the tube should always be checked by x-ray

11.5   Postoperative course and possible complications: Complementary measures

The lethality rate after early surgery in acute necrotizing pancreatitis is high. This is not surprising if we bear in mind that only patients who had little chance of survival after unsuccessful exclusively conservative prior treatment undergo operations. The early postoperative course, furthermore, requires the whole array of active internistic therapy under intensive interdisciplinary surveillance. Metabolic disorders (transitory or permanent diabetes) are to be expected after extensive pancreatic surgery such as removal or resection of the pancreas because of underlying necrosis.

Leading general postoperative complications in the order of incidence are: bronchopulmonary infections, wound infections, pancreatic fistulas, defective wound healing (wound rupture, abdominal wall rupture), hematemesis (due to stress bleeding), peripancreatic abscesses, and postoperative ileus due to adhesions [206, 210, 211, 212, 213].

Of all complications, postoperative fistulas have the best chances of healing spontaneously.

11.6   Delayed operation

Once the acute phase of an acute necrotizing pancreatitis has been overcome, delayed complications may develop from the autodigestive inflammatory process or occur locally. The clinical picture and the symptomatology are determined by the anatomically predestined encapsulated situation of the organ in the retroperitoneal bursa. This also accounts for an occasional seemingly paradoxical disease course in such cases and in patients who, having less extensive necrosis, survive the acute stage initially and then develop, or succumb to, grave complications in the further course. Renewed pain, rising body temperatures, and leukocytosis with suspicious palpation findings are the principal clinical symptoms. An optimal diagnostic workup with repeated sonography in addition to computed tomography, as outlined in Chapter 6, is indispensable. The formation of pseudocysts is one of the relatively most favorable postacute complications. If the walls are susceptible to anastomosis, the pseudocysts can be linked up with internal anastomoses to the upper small intestine. Initially delayed surgery in hemorrhagic-necrotizing pancreatitis is associated with an average mortality rate of 39%, according to the experience of the Mainz Pancreatic Center and Kümmerle's study group [258, 259, 340].

11.7   Summary

In closing, we should call attention especially to the fact that in the presence of a severe hemorrhagic-necrotizing pancreatitis a second operation and possibly several additional operations are unavoidable, offering the only chance and the last recourse. This is true if the first intervention has been scheduled too early and it is found that the pathological changes are not as yet sufficiently delineated to allow an exeresis or removal of necrotic tissue to be performed with adequate precision. A second operation is frequently necessitated also by the subsequent appearance of pancreatic sequestra, by their superinfection, or by progression of necrosis in a pancreatic segment which still appeared normal at the time of the first operation. The onset of late abscesses requires a third intervention in some cases.

Pending the availability of conclusive pathogenetic data on acute pancreatitis, an etiologically or causally oriented surgical treatment is possible only in the presence of pathological biliary tract changes due to lithiasis and inflammation. Of necessity, we have to be content with a certain empiricism consistent with each individual case in all forms of pancreatitis. The foremost guiding principle should therefore be: as early as possible, and doing as little harm as possible.

Two rules ought to govern all surgical-therapeutic endeavors:

Treat the patient, not only the pancreas!
Do what you can, not what you like!

Chapter 12 – Measures to be Taken Immediately when Acute Pancreatitis is Suspected

Only an early initiation of therapy can benefit the course and prognosis of acute pancreatitis!

The most important diagnostic and therapeutic measures to be taken in acute pancreatitis are summarized in Table 34. Every patient in whom acute pancreatitis is suspected has to be referred at once to a hospital where a quick diagnosis, intensive monitoring, and the application of appropriate therapeutic measures are assured. The most pressing action to be taken, even before the patient's transfer to the hospital, is pain relief (e.g., pentazocine; beware of morphine!) (see 10.1). In the presence of symptoms of hypovolemic shock, appropriate infusion therapy taking fluid, protein, and electrolyte losses into account (e.g., pancreatic edema, protein-rich exudate, ileus) (see Chapter 3) is of prime importance (glucose, electrolyte, and human albumin solutions in physiological concentrations). When dextran solutions are used, their effect on coagulation has to be considered.

At the *hospital,* the presumptive diagnosis of acute pancreatitis has to be quickly confirmed (lipase or amylase, sonography, and if even possible CT), and differential diagnosis has to rule out other abdominal diseases as well as myocardial infarction (ECG, enzymes), which can simulate an acute abdomen (see Chapters 6 and 7). The general diagnostic and therapeutic measures for acute pancreatitis are summarized in Tables 29 and 30, Chapter 10. Laboratory investigations for evaluation of the disease course are shown in Table 20, Chapter 6, and in Table 24, Chapter 8. The prevention and detection of complications have to rely primarily on the monitoring of circulatory parameters (including measurement of CVP), urine output, serum electrolytes (particularly K^+ and Ca^{++}), albumin, creatinine, BUN, γ-CT, alkaline phosphatase, transaminases, LDH, CBC, serum glucose, blood gases, and coagulation indices.

Besides pain control, the replacement of fluid and electrolytes, possibly human albumin and blood, and strict abstention from oral food and fluid intake and nasogastric tube in suspected ileus and gastric atony are of the greatest therapeutic urgency (see Table 29, Chapter 10). Gastric acid secretion may be blocked by cimetidine or ranitidine as well as by pirenzepine. Hyperglycemia is treated by i.v. infusion (Perfusor!) of regular insulin (unmodified insulin) with cautious dosage and a careful check on blood sugar values.

Inasmuch as the disease course is frequently unpredictable at the time of the diagnosis (edematous or hemorrhagic-necrotizing pancreatitis), the use of drugs to *inhibit pancreatic secretion* (somatostatin, calcitonin) and of *protease inhibitors* is generally justified. In view of the pathogenetic and pathophysiological mechanisms involved, this treatment should be given *as soon as possible,* that is, immediately after the diagnosis.

Hollender [199] recommends the i.v. administration of 500,000 KIU of aprotinin (Trasylol®) as a short-term infusion followed by an infusion of 2,000,000 KIU of aprotinin in 24 hours (preferably via a central venous catheter to avoid vein irritation). This treatment may conceivably have a favorable effect on shock symptoms that have already set in.

130

If merely "obscure upper abdominal pain" is present, aprotinin, somatostatin, or calcitonin are not indicated, not even in patients with mild episodes of an advanced chronic relapsing pancreatitis.

Validation of the diagnosis should be accompanied by the search for possible *etiological factors* (see Chapters 2 and 6: concerning history, e.g., cholelithiasis, chronic alcoholism, drugs; laboratory investigations, e.g., hyperparathyroidism, hyperlipoproteinemia; sonography, e.g., cholecystolithiasis, stasis in bile duct system, choledocholithiasis). In cases of biliary reflux pancreatitis due to choledocholithiasis and an obstruction in the bile duct system, an *endoscopic papillotomy* should be performed out immediately after the diagnosis (sonography!); if this should fail, surgical intervention has to follow (see Chapters 10 and 11).

If there already is evidence of intraabdominal exudation ("ascites"), *therapeutic peritoneal lavage* (peritoneal dialysis) should be considered besides the diagnostic one.

With respect to the diagnosis and therapy of complications, the pertinent chapters may be consulted. It should be stressed that dialysis must be instituted early in the presence of incipient renal failure (decrease of urine output, increased levels of creatinine and BUN). In incipient respiratory insufficiency, too, an early assisted or controlled ventilation with PEEP (positive end-expiratory pressure) has to be initiated. At the same time a causal treatment should be administered if possible (e.g., surgical removal of the septic focus originating in pancreas).

Every acute pancreatitis as well as every severe attack of a chronic relapsing pancreatitis calls for intensive interdisciplinary management – to be instituted immediately after diagnosis – particularly in terms of joint continuous surveillance of the patient (local findings, general condition, laboratory investigations, sonography, CT) so that the decision to operate may be made jointly by the surgeon and the internist, and this at the "optimal" time.

Surgical intervention (when indicated to save the patient's life) is a necessity if the disease course worsens despite maximal, intensive conservative therapy and, specifically, if symptoms of shock persist, necrosis spreads, abscesses form, and sepsis as well as renal or respiratory insufficiency develops (see Chapter 11).

Family physician / emergency physician:
Hospital (intensive care unit):
Conservative therapy:
Indications for surgical therapy:

Table 34. Immediate
diagnostic and therapeutic
measures
in acute pancreatitis

- Pain relief (see Chapter 10.1; beware of morphine!)
- Possible initiation of shock therapy (human albumin, electrolyte or glucose solution in physiological concentration)
- Immediate hospitalization

- Surveillance of patient (see Chapter 10, specifically Table 30), particularly circulatory, renal, and pulmonary function, fluid and electrolyte balance, local abdominal changes
- Confirmation of diagnosis (lipase or amylase, sonography, and if even possible, CT, diagnostic peritoneal lavage; see Chapter 6), differential diagnosis (see Chapter 7)

- General therapeutic measures, e.g., pain control, fluid and electrolyte replacement (check balance, CVP), possibly human albumin, blood; no food or fluids by mouth; in ileus: nasogastric tube (see Chapter 10, specifically Table 29)
- Administration of protease inhibitors (aprotinin, Trasylol®) and/or drugs to inhibit pancreatic and gastric secretion (e.g., somatostatin, calcitonin, H_2-blockers, pirenzepine)
- Therapeutic peritoneal lavage
- Exploration of etiological factors; causal therapy if possible (e.g., endoscopic papillotomy in biliary reflux pancreatitis)
- Antibiotics (e.g., in biliary pancreatitis, cholangitis, suspected sepsis)
- Prevention or early treatment of complications (shock: see above; renal insufficiency: dialysis; diabetes: unmodified insulin iv (Perfusor!); respiratory insufficiency: early assisted or controlled ventilation with positive end-expiratory pressure (PEEP)

- Failure of endoscopic papillotomy for treatment of biliary reflux pancreatitis
- Exacerbation of disease course despite exhaustive conservative therapy, persistent shock, renal failure, secondary in spread of necrosis, sequestration, abscess formation, onset of additional complications (e.g., respiratory insufficiency, ileus)

References

1. Abcarian, H., Eftaiha, M., Kraft, A. R., and Nyhus, L. M.: Colonic complications of acute pancreatitis. Arch. Surg. 114: 995, 1979.
2. Achord, J. L.: Acute pancreatitis with infectious hepatitis. JAMA 205: 837, 1968.
3. Acosta, J. M., and Ledesma, C. L.: Gallstone migration as a cause of acute pancreatitis. New Eng. J. Med. 290: 484, 1974.
4. Acosta, J. M. Pellegrini, C. A., and Skinner, D. B.: Etiology and pathogenesis of acute biliary pancreatitis. Surgery 88: 118, 1980.
5. Alexandre, J. H., Camilleri, J. P., Assan, R., Guerrieri, M. T., and Bonan, A.: Indications et résultats de la pancréatectomie totale dans le traitement des pancréatites aiguës nécrosantes. Chirurgie 103: 858, 1977.
6. Alexandre, J. H., Chambon, H., and Assan, R.: Total pancreatectomy in the treatment of acute necrotizing and hemorrhagic pancreatitis. Langenbeck's Arch. klin. Chir. 340: 231, 1976.
7. Alexandre, J. H., and Germain, M.: La nécrose colique au cours de pancréatites aiguës. Ann. Chir. 26: 857, 1972.
8. Allison, A. C.: Lysosomes in disease. Science J. 1: 32, 1965.
9. Ammann, R.: Acute pancreatitis. In: H. L. Bockus (Ed.): Gastroenterology, Vol. 3, 3rd ed. Saunders (Philadelphia, Eastbourne, Toronto), 1976.
10. Amundsen, E.: The clinical significance of proteinase inhibitors. Acta Chir. Scand., Suppl. 378: 111, 1967.
11. Amundsen, E.: Pathophysiologische Problematik der akuten Pankreatitis. Leber, Magen, Darm 6: 199, 1977.
12. Amundsen, E.: Pathophysiologie der akuten Pankreatitis. In: H. Sarles and M. Singer (Eds.): Akute und chronische Pankreatitis. Witzstrock (Baden-Baden, Cologne, New York), 1978.
13. Amundsen, E., Ofstad, E., and Hagen, P. O.: Experimental acute pancreatitis in dogs. 1. Hypotensive effect induced by pancreatic exudate. Scand. J. Gastroent. 3: 659, 1968.
14. Anand, S. S., Sotantar, R., and Pathok, I. C.: Experimental production of acute pancreatitis in dogs by duct obstruction. Indian H. Surg. 22: 261, 1960.
15. Anam-Sefat, J. C., Blair, E., and Reckler, S.: Primary mesenteric venous occlusive disease. S.G.O. 141: 740, 1975.
16. Anderson, M. C.: Pathophysiology of acute pancreatitis. Invited commentary. World J. Surg. 5: 325, 1981.
17. Anderson, M. C., Needlemann, S. B., Gramatica, L., Toranto, I. R., and Briggs, D. R.: Further inquiry into the pathogenesis of acute pancreatitis. Role of pancreatic enzymes. Arch. Surg. 99: 185, 1969.
18. Anderson, M. C., and Schiller, W. R.: Microcirculatory dynamics in the normal and inflamed pancreas. Amer. J. Surg. 115: 118, 1968.
19. Arbeiter, B., Marsch-Ziegler, U., Leonhardt, H., and Schäfer, J.-H.: Retrospektive Erhebungen zum Wert der Laparoskopie bei der Differenzierung von akuter edematöser und akuter hämorrhagisch-nekrotisierender Pankreatitis in der Frühphase der Erkrankung. Z. Gastroent. 19: 173, 1981.
20. Arnesjö, B.: Pancreatic phospholipase. Physiological chemistry and possible aetiologic role in acute pancreatitis. Thesis, University of Lund, 1968.
21. Arnesjö, B., and Grubb, B. A.: Intracellular distribution of lipase in comparison to trypsinogen, amylase and immediately measurable trypsin inhibitor(s) in the rat pancreas. Acta Physiol. Scand. 75: 139, 1969.
22. Arnold, F., Doyle, P. J., and Bell, G.: Acute pancreatitis in a patient treated with cimetidine. Lancet I: 382, 1978.
23. Autio, V., Juusela, E., and Lauslahti, K.: Resection of the pancreas for acute hemorrhagic and necrotizing pancreatitis. World J. Surg. 3: 631, 1979.
24. Babb, R. R.: The role of surgery in acute pancreatitis. Dig. Dis. Sci. 21: 672, 1976.
25. Back, N.: Death from acute pancreatitis. Lancet II: 370, 1978.

26. Bagdade, J. D.: Diabetic lipaemia complicating acute pancreatitis. Lancet 7629, 1041, 1969.

27. Baldwin, W. M.: Pancreatic ducts in man, together with a study of the microscopical structure of the minor duodenal papilla. Anat. Rec. 5: 197, 1911.

28. Balldin, G.: On protease-antiprotease imbalance with special reference to the protective role of protease inhibitors in acute pancreatitis. Akademisk Avhandling, Malmö, 1980.

29. Balldin, G., Gustafson, E.-L., and Ohlsson, K: Influence of plasma proteae inhibitors and Trasylol on trypsin-induced bradykinin relase. Eur. Surg. Res. 12: 260, 1980.

30. Balldin, G., Laurell, C.-B., and Ohlsson, K.: Increased catabolism of α-macroglubulins after intravenous infusion of trypsin-α_1-antitrypsin complexes in dogs. Hoppe-Seylers Z. Physiol. Chem. 359: 699, 1978.

31. Balldin, G., and Ohlsson, K.: Demonstration of pancreatic protease-antiprotease complexes in the peritoneal fluid of patients with acute pancreatitis. Surgery 85: 451, 1979.

32. Balldin, G., and Ohlsson, K.: Trasylol prevents trypsin-induced shocks in dogs. Hoppe-Seylers Z. Physiol. Chem. 360: 651, 1979.

33. Balldin, G., Ohlsson, K., and Ohlsson, A.-S.: Studies on the influence of Trasylol on the partition of trypsin between the human plasma protease inhibitors in vitro. Hoppe-Seylers Z. Physiol. Chem. 359: 691, 1978.

34. Banks, S., and Marks, I. N.: Case reports, hyperlipemic pancreatitis and the pill. Postgrad. Med. J. 46: 576, 1970.

35. Bartelheimer, H.: Klinik der akuten und chronischen Pankreatitis. Verh. dtsch. Ges. inn. Med. 70: 759, 1964.

36. Bartelheimer, H., Classen, M., and Ossenberg, F. W.: Die Behandlung der kranken Bauchspeicheldrüse. II. Hamburger medizinisches Symposium. Thieme, 1978.

37. Bauer-Hack, K.: Ovulationshemmer und Pankreopathie. Med. Welt 21: 1739, 1970.

38. Beck, I. Th., Kahn, D. S., Solymar, J. McKenna, R. D., and Zylberszac, B.: The role of pancreatic enzymes in the pathologic and biochemical changes in the canine pancreas to intraductal injection with bile and with trypsin. Gastroenterology 46: 531, 1964.

39. Becker, H., Ruf, W., Hissen, E., and Junghanns, K.: A prospective study to determine the efficacy of dextran 40 in acute pancreatitis. In: L. F. Hollender (Ed.), Controversies in acute pancreatitis. Springer (Berlin–Heidelberg–New York), 1982.

40. Becker, V.: Sekretionsstudien am Pankreas. Thieme (Stuttgart), 1957.

41. Becker, V.: Bauchspeicheldrüse. In: Doerr–Seifert–Uehlinger: Spezielle pathologische Anatomie, Vol. 6. Springer (Berlin–Heidelberg–New York), 1973.

42. Becker, V., and Wilde, W.: Pankreasschäden durchTrypsin in vitro. Klin. Wschr. 41: 73, 1963.

43. Bell, E. T.: Pancreatitis. Surgery 43: 527, 1958.

44. Ben Abdeljlil, A.: Enzymadaption des exokrinen Pankreas auf Nahrung und hormonale Reize. Z. Gastroent. 4: 235, 1966.

45. Blackburn, G. L., Maini, B. S., and Pierce, E. C.: Nutrition in the critically ill patient. Anesthesiology 47: 181, 1977.

46. Bleyl, U.: Die sogenannte nervale Pankreatitis und ihre pathophysiologischen Grundlagen. Z. Gastroent. 1: 335, 1963.

47. Bleyl, U., Grözinger, K.-H., Nagel, W., and Wanke, M.: Histochemische Darstellung proteolytischer Aktivität bei der akuten experimentellen Pankreatitis. Klin. Wschr. 44: 282, 1966.

48. Bleyl, U., Grözinger, K.-H., Nagel, W., and Wanke, M.: Histotopochemie aktiver proteolytischer Enzyme bei der experimentellen autodigestiven Pankreatitis. Virchows Arch. path. Anat. 342: 26, 1967.

49. Bleyl, U., and Wanke, M.: Morphologische und gerinnungsanalytische Untersuchungen zum postpankreatitischen Schock. In: G. L. Haberland and P. Matis (Eds.): Neue Aspekte der Trasyloltherapie 3, p. 111. Schattauer (Stuttgart–New York), 1969.

50. Block, F.: Der Verdauungstrakt und die großen Drüsen. In: Büchner–Letterer–Roulet: Handbuch der allgemeinen Pathologie, Vol. III/2, p. 277. Springer (Berlin–Göttingen–Heidelberg), 1960.

51. Bode, J. Ch., and Dürr, H. K.: Therapie der akuten Pankreatitis. In: H. Sarles and M. Singer (Eds.): Akute und chronische Pankreatitis. Witzstrock (Baden-Baden, Cologne, New York), 1978.

52. Bolooki, H., and Gliedmann, M. L.: Peritoneal dialysis in treatment of acute pancreatitis. Surgery 64: 466, 1968.

53. Borgström, B.: Hydrolysis and synthesis of glyceride ester bonds catalyzed by pancreatic lipase. Biochim. Biophys. Acta 84: 228, 1964.

54. Boumghar, M., and Cavin, R.: Respiratorische Komplikationen bei schwerer akuter Pankreatitis. Schweiz. Rundschau Med. 67: 1394, 1978.

55. Bourne, M. S., and Dawson, H.: Acute pancreatitis complicating prednisolone therapy. Lancet 7058, 1209, 1958.

56. Boutelier, P.: Les indications opératoires précoces dans les pancréatites aigües. Ann. Chir. 26: 261, 1972.

57. Boutelier, P., and Edelmann, G.: Tactique chirurgicale dans les pancréatites aigües nécrosantes. Plaidoyer en faveur des sequestrectomies. Ann. Chir. 26: 249, 1972.

58. Brodehl, J.: Pankreatitis durch experimentelle Allergie. Scient. Meeting of North and West German Pathologists. Zbl. allg. Path. path. Anat. 100: 356, 1959.

59. Brodrick, J. W., Geokas, M. C., Largman, C., Fasset, M., and Johnson, J. H.: Molecular forms of immunoreactive cationic trypsin in pancreatitis patient sera. Am. J. Physiol. 237: E 474, 1979.

60. Brodrick, J. W., Largman, C., Ray, S. B., and Geokas, M. C.: Proteolysis of parathyroid hormone in vitro by sera from acute pancreatitis patients. Proc. Soc. Exp. Biol. Med. 167: 588, 1981.

61. Brunzell, J. D., and Schrott, H. G.: Interaction of familial and secondary causes of hypertriglyceridemia: Role in pancreatitis. Clin. Res. 21: 723, 1973.

62. Bücheler, E., Montgomery, F. U., and Grabbe, E.: Röntgendiagnostik des Pankreas. Internist 23: 82, 1982.

63. Büchner, F.: Allgemeine Pathologie. Urban & Schwarzenberg (Munich–Berlin), 1950.

64. Büchner, F.: Stoffwechsel und Struktur. Prolegomena einer allgemeinen Pathologie. In: Handbuch der allgemeinen Pathologie, Vol. I. Springer (Berlin–Heidelberg–New York), 1969.

65. Bünte, H.: Pankreatitis nach Magenresektion. Langenbecks Arch. Chir. 329: 1054, 1971.

66. Budd, G. C., Darzynkiewicz, A., and Barnard, E. A.: Intracellular localization of specific proteases in rat mast cells. Nature (London) 213: 1202, 1967.

67. Cameron, J. L. Capuzzi, D. M., and Zuidema, G. D.: Acute pancreatitis with hyperlipemia. Amer. J. Med. 56: 482, 1974.

68. Cameron, J. L., Megikan, D., and Zuidema, G. D.: Evaluation of atropine in acute pancreatitis. Surgery 148: 206, 1979.

69. Carey, L. C.: Extra-abdominal manifestations of acute pancreatitis. Surgery 86: 337, 1979.

70. Cattel, R. B., and Warren, K. W.: Surgery of the pancreas. W. B. Saunders Co. (Philadelphia–London), 1953.

71. Champetier, J., Bouchet, Y., Brahant, A., Guignier, M., Durant, A., Charignon, G., and Corallo, J.: L'extension au côlon de la nécrose pancréatique. Trois observations. Lyon Chir. 70: 196, 1974.

72. Charleux, H., Mongredien, Ph., Anfroy, J. P., Normand, P., and Fichelle, A.: A propos de "la non-fermenture pariétale" dans la chirurgie des péritonites. Chirurgie 106: 63, 1980.

73. Clavadetscher, P., and Weber, H.: Klinische Nebenwirkungen und biochemische Veränderungen unter Ovulationshemmern. Schweiz. med. Wschr. 103: 231, 1973.

74. Colin, R., Lapeyrie, H., and Dossa, J.: La pancréatectomie précoce dans les pancréatites aigües nécrotiques. Mém. Acad. Chir. 94: 437, 1968.

75. Coltmant, H. J., and Noltenius, H.: Pankreatische Enzephalopathie. Med. Klin. 72: 2146, 1977.

76. Comfort, M. W., and Steinberg, A. G.: Pedigree of a family with hereditary chronic relapsing pancreatitis. Gastroenterology 21: 54, 1952.

77. Cooperman, M., Ferrara, J. J., Carey, L. C., Thomas, F. B., Martin, E. W., Jr., and Fromkes, J. J.: Idiopathic acute pancreatitis: The value of endoscopie retrograde cholangiopancreatography. Surgery 90: 666, 1981.

78. Cotton, P. B.: Endoscopie retrograde pancreaticography. In: H. T. Howat, and H. Sarles (Eds.): The exocrine pancreas. Saunders (London–Philadelphia–Toronto), 1979.

79. Cox, A. G.: Death from acute pancreatitis: M.R.C. Multicenter trial of glucagon and aprotinin. Lancet II: 632, 1977.

80. Creutzfeldt, W.: Kininfreisetzung bei Pankreatitis. In: Neue Aspekte der Trasyloltherapie III, p. 89. Schattauer (Stuttgart–New York), 1969.

81. Creutzfeldt, W.: Erkrankungen der Bauchspeicheldrüse. In: R. Gross and P. Schölmerich (Eds.): Lehrbuch der inneren Medizin, 3rd ed. Schattauer, 1982.

82. Creutzfeldt, W., and Lankisch, P. G.: Intensive medical treatment of severe acute pancreatitis. World J. Surg. 5: 341, 1981.

83. Creutzfeldt, W., and Schmidt, H.: Aetiology and pathogenesis of pancreatitis. Scand. J. Gastroent. 5 (Suppl. 6): 47, 1970.

84. Cross, D. F.: Recurrent pancreatitis and fat-induced hyperlipoproteinemia. JAMA 8: 1494, 1969.

85. Cross, K. R.: Accessory pancreatic ducts. Special reference to the intrapancreatic portion of the common duct. Arch. Path. 62: 434, 1956.

86. Dagnini, G.: What can be expected of laparoscopy in the diagnosis of acute pancreatitis. In: L. F. Hollender (Ed.): Controversies in acute pancreatitis. Springer (Berlin–Heidelberg–New York), 1982.

87. Dammann, H. G.: Komplikationen der akuten Pankreatitis. Pathogenese, Therapie und Prognose. Med. Klin. 73: 1029, 1978.

88. Dammann, H. G.: Akute hämorrhagisch-nekrotisierende Pankreatitis. Med. Klin. 76: 186, 1981.

89. Damman, H. G., Döpner, M., v. Wichert, L., and Harders, H.: Die Beurteilung der Frühprognose der akuten Pankeatitis. Zbl. Chir. 106: 154, 1981.

90. Dammann, H. G., Grabbe, E., and Flashoff, D.: Klinische laborchemische und computertomographische Charakterisierung des vital bedrohten Patienten bei akuter Pankreatitis. Leber, Magen, Darm 11: 174, 1981.

91. Dammann, H. G., v. Wichert, P., and Schreiber, H. W.: Prognostische Indizes bei der akuten Pankreatitis. Eine retrospektive Studie. Zbl. Chir. 104: 397, 1979.

92. Darzynkiewicz, A., and Barnard, E. A.: Specific proteases of the rat mast cell. Nature (London) 213: 1198, 1967.

93. Deenen, L. L. M., van: Phospholipids and biomembranes. In: R. T. Holman (Ed.): Progress in the chemistry of fats and other lipids. Pergamon Press (London), 1965.

94. De Haas, G. H., Postema, N. M., Nieuwenhuizen, W., and van Deenen, L. M.: Purification and properties of phosholipase A from porcine pancreas. Biochim. Biophys. Acta 159: 103, 1968.

95. Delany, H. M., Carnavale, N., and Garvey, J. W.: Jejunostomy by needle catheter technique. Surgery 73: 786, 1973.

96. Delany, H. M., Carnavale, N., Garvey, J. W., and Moss, C. M.: Postoperative nutritional support using needle catheter feeding jejunostomy. Ann. Surg. 186: 165, 1977.

97. Desnuelle, P.: Adaptation der Enzyme des exokrinen Pankreas aus der Sicht der Biosynthese. Z. Gastroent. 4: 236, 1966.

98. Desnuelle, P., and Figarella, C.: Biochemistry. In: H. T. Howat and H. Sarles (Eds.): The exocrine pancreas. Saunders (London–Philadelphia–Toronto), 1979.

99. DiMagno, E. P.: What is appropriate non-operative treatment of acute pancreatitis? Dig. Dis. Sci. 24: 337, 1979.

100. Doerr, W.: Pankreatitis, Pathogenese, Formen, Häufigkeit. Langenbecks Arch. klin. Chir. 292: 552, 1959.

101. Doerr, W., Diezel, P. B., Grözinger, K.-H., Lasch, H. G., Nagel, W., Rossner, J. R., Wanke, M., and Willig, F.: Pathogenese der experimentellen autodigestiven Pankreatitis. Klin. Wschr. 43: 125, 1965.

102. Donath, K., Mitschke, H., and Seifert, G.; Ultrastrukturelle Veränderungen am Rattenpankreas beim hämorrhagischen Schock. Beitr. Path. 141: 33, 1970.

103. Duerr, G. H. K.: Acute pancreatitis. In: H. T. Howat and H. Sarles (Eds.): The exocrine pancreas. Saunders (London), 1979.

104. Dürr, H. K.: Alkoholschädigung des Pankreas. Internist 19: 123, 1978.

105. Dürr, H. K., and Bode, J. Ch.: Klinik und Therapie der akuten Pankreatitis. Leber, Magen, Darm 6: 282, 1976.

106. Dürr. H. K., Maroske, D., Zelder, O., and Bode, J. Ch.: Glucagon therapy in acute pancreatitis. Gut 19: 175, 1978.

107. Eckert, P., Riesner, K., and Doehn, M.: Indikationen zur Therapie mit Proteinasehemmern in der Chirurgie. Med. Welt 25: 2154, 1974.

108. Edelmann, G., and Boutelier, P.: Le traitement des pancréatites aiguës nécrosantes par l'ablation chirurgicale précoce des portions nécrosantes. Mém. Acad. Chir. 100: 155, 1974.

109. Editorial: Ultrasonography of the pancreas. Lancet II: 1212, 1979.

110. Ehrlich, E. W., Howard, J. M., and Spitzer, J. J.: Lipid disturbances in pancreatitis with reference to hyperlipemia

in the acute stage. Clin. Res. 7: 368, 1960.

111. Eiseman, B., Beart, R., and Norton, L.: Multiple organ failure. Surg. Gynec. Obstet. 144: 323, 1977.

112. Evander, A., and Ihse, I.: Cimetidine treatment in acute experimental pancreatitis. Eur. Surg. Res. 12: 301, 1980.

113. Fagniez, P. L., Hay, J. M., Regnier, B., Maillard, J. N., Julien, M., Germain, A., and Elman, A.: Péritonites "dépassées". Attitudes thérapeutiques et résultats. Nouv. Presse Méd. 8: 1348, 1979.

114. Fagniez, P. L., Julien, M., Velluet, M., and Germain, A.: Sur le traitement chirurgical des pancréatites aiguës nécrosantes. A propos de 47 cas. Chirurgie 100: 816, 1974.

115. Fahrtmann, E. H., and Männl, H. F. K.: Postoperative Pankreatitis – Übersicht. In: Aktuelle Chirurgie: Die Chirurgie der akuten und chronischen Pankreatitis. TM-Verlag 1980, Berlin Symposium.

116. Farmer, R. G., Kinkelman, E. I., Brown, H. B., and Lewis, L. A.: Hyperlipoproteinemia and pancreatitis. Amer. J. Med. 54: 161, 1973.

117. Farnan, L. W.: Pancreatitis following mumps. Report of case with operation. Amer. J. Med. Sci. 163: 859, 1922.

118. Ferner, H.: Das hyperglykämisierende Prinzip des Pankreas, sowie über Gefäßverhältnisse und Innervation der Inseln. Acta Neuroveg. (Vienna) 9: 47, 1954.

119. Ferner, H.: Über hormonale Nahwirkung. Die Dissemination endokriner Zellgruppen als funktionelles Prinzip. Dtsch. med. Wschr. 83: 1468, 1958.

120. Figarella, C., Clemente, F., and Guy, E.: On zymogens of human pancreatic juice. FEBS Letters 3: 351, 1969.

121. Fikry, M.: Exocrine pancreatic functions in the aged. J. Amer. Geriat. Soc. 16: 463, 1968.

122. Finley, J. W.: Respiratory complications of acute pancreatitis. Amer. J. Surg. 35: 591, 1969.

123. Flament, J. B., Pluot, M., Convers, G., Delattre, J. F., and Rives, J.: Nécrose colique au cours de la pancréatite aiguë nécrotico-hémorrhagique. Méd. Chir. Dig. 10: 31, 1981.

124. Frey, C. F.: Hemorrhagic pancreatitis. Amer. J. Surg. 137: 616, 1979.

125. Frey, Ch. F., Hin Nang Wong, Hickmann, D., and Pullos, T.: Toxicity of hemorrhagic ascitic fluid associated with hemorrhagic pancreatitis. Arch. Surg. 117: 401, 1982.

126. Fritsch, A., Lechner, G., and Zaunbauer, W.: Klinische und angiographische Untersuchungen bei Verschlußkrankheit der großen Eingeweidearterien. Int. Surg. 57: 381, 1972.

127. Forell, M. M., and Lehnert, P.: Physiologie und Biochemie von Verdauung und Resorption: Verdauung. In: H.-D. Cremer, D. Hötzel and J. Kühnau (Eds.): Ernährungslehre und Diätetik, ein Handbuch in vier Bänden. Vol. I, Part 1, Biochemie und Physiologie der Ernährung. Thieme (Stuttgart–New York), 1980.

128. Forell, M. M., and Lehnert, P.: Gallenwege und exokrines Pankreas. In: W. Siegenthaler (Ed.): Klinische Pathophysiologie, 5th ed. Thieme (Stuttgart–New York), 1982.

129. Forell, M. M., and Lehnert, P.: Anomalien und entzündliche Erkrankungen des Pankreas. In: H. Hornbostel, W. Kaufmann, and W. Siegenthaler (Eds.): Innere Medizin in Praxis und Klinik, Vol. IV, Verdauungstrakt, Ernährungsstörungen, Stoffwechsel, Vergiftungen, 3rd ed. Thieme (Stuttgart–New York), 1983 (in press).

130. Forell, M. M., Stahlheber, H., and Fritz, H.: Zur Frage der trypsinhemmenden Wirkung des Duodenalsaftes. Klin. Wschr. 43: 1007, 1965.

131. Forell, M. M., Stahlheber, H., Lehnert, P., Londong, W., Teufel, H., Fritz, H., and Roder, O.: Physiologie des exokrinen Pankreas, In: M. M. Forell (Ed.): Handbuch der inneren Medizin, 5th ed., Vol. 3/5. Springer (Berlin–Heidelberg–New York), 1976.

132. Forell, M. M., Stahlheber, H., and Scholz, F.: Galle als Reiz der Enzymsekretion des Pankreas. Dtsch. med. Wschr. 90: 1128, 1965.

133. Fredrickson, D. S., Goldstein, J. L., and Brown, M. S.: The familiar hyperlipoproteinemias, 4th ed., New York, 1978.

134. Frey, E. K., Kraut, H., and Werle, E.: Das Kallikrein-Kinin-System und seine Inhibitoren, 2nd ed. Enke (Stuttgart), 1968.

135. Fritz, H., Fink, E., and Trutscheit, E.: Kallikrein inhibitors. Fed. Proc. 38: 2753, 1979.

136. Fritz, H., Hutzel, M., Hüller, I., Wiedemann, M., Stahlheber, H., Lehnert, P., and Forell, M. M.: Über das Sekretionsverhalten der spezifischen Trypsininhibitoren und des Kallikreinogens beim Pankreas von Hund und

Mensch. Hoppe-Seylers Z. Physiol, Chem. 348: 1575, 1967.

137. Fritz, H., Kruck, J., Rüsse, I., and Liebich, H. G.: Immunofluorescene studies indicate that the basic trypsin-kallikrein inhibitor of bovine organs (Trasylol) originates from mast cells. Hoppe-Seylers Z. Physiol. Chem. 360: 437, 1979.

138. Frosch, N., Wanke, M., Barth, P., and Wegener, K.: Hyperparathyreotische Krise mit Pankreatitis und subakuter Leberdystrophie. Dtsch. med. Wschr. 90: 1039, 1965.

139. Fuller, R. K., Loveland, J. P., and Frankel, M. H.: An evaluation of nasogastric suction treatment in alcoholic pancreatitis. Amer. J. Gastroenterol. 75: 349, 1981.

140. Fulton, M. C., and Marriott, H. L.: Acute pancreatitis simulating myocardial infarction. Ann. Int. 59: 730, 1963.

141. Gabryelewicz, A., Dlugosz, J., Brzozowski, J., Triebling, A., Werescynska, U., and Musiatowicz, B.: Effect of prostacyclin (PGI_1) on pancreatic lysosomes in acute experimental pancreatitis (AEP) in dogs. Digestion 25 (1): 34, 1982.

142. Gall, F.: Private communication, 1982.

143. Gauthier, A., Escoffier, J. M., Camatte, R., and Sarles, H.: Severe acute pancreatitis. Clin. Gastroenterol. 10: 209, 1981.

144. Gebauer, A., and Scherer, U.: Differentialindikation für die Computertomographie und die Ultraschalluntersuchung. Internist 19: 568, 1978.

145. Geiger, V.: Morphogenese der postnekrotischen Pankreaszirrhose. Doctoral thesis, Heidelberg, 1968.

146. Geokas, M. C., Murphy, D. R., and McKenna, R. D.: The role of elastase in acute pancreatitis. I. Intrapancreatic elastolytic activity in bileinduced acute pancreatitis in dogs. Arch. Path. 86: 117, 1968.

147. Geokas, M. C., Olsen, H., and Carmack, C.: Peritoneal lavage in the treatment of acute hemorrhagic pancreatitis. Gastroenterology 58: 950, 1970.

148. Geokas, M. C., and Rinderknecht, H.: Determination of methemalbumin in serum. In: M. M. Forell (Ed.): Handbuch der inneren Medizin, 5th ed., Vol. 3, Verdauungsorgane, Part 6, Pankreas. Springer (Berlin–Heidelberg–New York), 1976.

149. Geokas, M. C., Rinderknecht, H., Walberg, C. B., and Weissman, R.: Methemalbumin in the diagnosis of acute hemorrhagic pancreatitis. Ann. Intern. Med. 81: 483, 1974.

150. Gerhardt, Ch., and Stolte, M.: Die Ausschaltung des exkretorischen Pankreas-Parenchyms durch intraduktale Injektion einer schnell härtenden Aminosäurelösung. Chirurg 49: 428, 1978.

151. Gjone, E., Oestad, E., Marton, P., and Amundsen, E.: Phospholipase activity in pancreatic exudate in experimental acute pancreatitis. Scand. J. Gastroent. 2: 181, 1967.

152. Gmaz-Nikulin, E., Nikulin, A., and Plamenac, P.: Pancreatic lesions in shock and their significance. J. Path. (Edinburgh) 135: 223, 1981.

153. Göber, I.: Die Auswirkung des hypovolämischen Schocks auf das Pankreas. Wien. klin. Wschr. 87: 3, 1975.

154. Göbiet, J.: Beiträge zur operativen Behandlung der akuten und chronischen Pankreatitis. Wien. klin. Wschr. 23: 1672, 1910.

155. Goebell, H.: Diagnostische Möglichkeiten mit der Bestimmung von Amylase und Lipase in Körperflüssigkeiten. Internist 11: 117, 1970.

156. Goebell, H.: Was ist gesichert in der Therapie der akuten Pankreatitis? Internist 19: 700, 1978.

157. Goebell, H., Ammann, R., Herfarth, Ch., Horn, J., Hotz, J., Knoblauch, M., Schmid, M., Jaeger, M., Akovbiantz, A., Lindner, E., Abt, K., Nüesch, E., and Barth, E. (The Pancreatitis Study Group): A double-blind trial of synthetic salmon calcitonin in the treatment of acute pancreatitis. Scand. J. Gastroent. 14: 881, 1979.

158. Goebell, H., and Dürr, H.-K.: Die akute Pankreatitis – Pro und Contra der modernen Therapie. Internist 22: 684, 1981.

159. Goebell, H., and Hotz, J.: Die Ätiologie der akuten Pankreatitis. In: M. M. Forell (Ed.): Handbuch der inneren Medizin, 5th ed., Vol. 3: Verdauungsorgane, Part 6: Pankreas. Springer (Berlin–Heidelberg–New York), 1976.

160. Goebell, H., and Hotz, J.: Ätiologie der akuten Pankreatitis. In: H. Sarles and M. Singer (Eds.): Akute und chronische Pankreatitis. Witzstrock (Baden-Baden, Cologne, New York), 1978.

161. Goebell, H., and Hotz, J.: Kalzium, Pankreassekretion und Pankreatitis. Leber, Magen, Darm 6: 211, 1976.
162. Goebell, H., and Singer, M. V.: Wirkung von Alkohol am menschlichen und tierischen Pankreas. Leber, Magen, Darm 8: 304, 1978.
163. Goldstein, D. A., Lach, F., and Massry, S. G.: Acute renal failure in patients with acute pancreatitis. Arch. Intern. Med. 136: 1363, 1976.
164. Grana, W., and Wise, L.: Role of emergency laparotomy in acute pancreatitis. Amer. J. Surg. 42: 128, 1976.
165. Grözinger, K.-H.: Hemmkörpertherapie der akuten Pankreatitis. Münch. med. Wschr. 122: 234, 1980.
166. Grözinger, K.-H., and Wanke, M.: Angeborene Fehlbildungen des Pankreas. In: M. M. Forell (Ed.): Handbuch der inneren Medizin, Vol. 3/6. Springer (Berlin–Heidelberg), 1976.
167. Grözinger, K.-H., Wanke, M., Hochberg, K., Schüler, H. W., Walter, S. I., Welsh, P., and Farnusch, D.: Serumenzymveränderungen bei der experimentellen Pankreatitis des Hundes. Z. ges. exp. Med. 140: 136, 1966.
168. Gross, F. S., Raffucci, F. L., Brackney, E. L., and Wangensteen, O. W.: Relationship of prolonged drainage of bile through pancreatic duct system to pancreatitis. Proc. Soc. Exp. Biol. (N.Y.) 90: 208, 1955.
169. Gruber, U. F.: Dextran: Biochemische Wirkung, ärztliche Überwachung und Laboratoriumskontrolle. In: R. Marx and H. A. Thies (Eds.): Kontrolle von Antithrombotica. XXIII. Hamburger Symposium über Blutgerinnung. Editiones Roche (Basle, Grenzach-Whylen), 1981.
170. Grunst, J., and Paumgartner, G.: Akute Pankreatitis-Klinik, Diagnose und internistische Therapie. Chirurg 51: 364, 1980.
171. Guivarc'H, M., Mouchet, A., and Marquand, J.: A propos de 33 pancréatites nécrosantes traitées per exérèse. Mém. Acad. Chir. 100: 891, 1974.
172. Guivarc'H, M., Roullet-Audy, J. C., and Chapmann, A.: La non-fermeture dans la chirurgie itérative des péritonites. Chirurgie 105: 287, 1979.
173. Gülzow, M.: Die eitrige Pankreatitis. Med. Klin. 51: 413, 1956.
174. Gülzow, M.: Pankreatitis durch Behandlung mit Kortikosteroiden (klinische und experimentelle Untersuchungen). Dtsch. Z. Verdau. Stoffwechselkr. 20: 168, 1960.
175. Güthert, H.: Pankreas. In: E. Kaufmann (Ed.): Handbuch der speziellen pathologischen Anatomie, Vol. II/2, p. 1334. De Gruyter (Berlin), 1958.
176. Haberland, G., and McConn, R.: A rationale for the therapeutic action of aprotinin. Fed. Proc. 38: 2760, 1979.
177. Haberland, G., and Matis, P.: Trasylol, ein Proteinaseninhibitor. Med. Welt 18: 1367, 1967.
178. Habermann, E.: Probleme der Pathophysiologie des Kininsystems. In: Neue Aspekte der Trasylol-Therapie III, p. 37. Schattauer (Stuttgart–New York), 1969.
179. Hallberg, D., and Theve, N. O.: Observations during treatment of acute pancreatitis with insulin and glucose infusions. Acta Chir. Scand. 140: 138, 1974.
180. Hardaway, R. M.: Syndromes of disseminated intravascular coagulation. Thomas (Springfield, Ill.), 1966.
181. Hartung, H., and Kirchner, R.: Diagnostik und Therapie der akuten Pankreatitis. Leber, Magen, Darm 10: 1, 1980.
182. Hay, J. M., Duchatelle, P., Elman, A., Flamant, Y., and Maillard, J. N.: Les ventres laissé ouverts. Chirurgie 105: 508, 1979.
183. Hayes, M. F., Rosenbaum, R. W., and Zibelman, M.: Adult respiratory distress syndrome in association with acute pancreatitis. Amer. J. Surg. 127: 314, 1974.
184. Heberer, M.: Jejunostomie. Klinikarzt 11: 1035, 1982.
185. Heldwein, W., and Lehnert, P.: Unpublished results.
186. Hess, W.: Die chronische Pankreatitis. Huber (Berne–Stuttgart), 1969.
187. Hodgson, H. J. F., Whitaker, K. B., Cooper, B. T., Baron, J. H., Freeman, H. G. M., Moos, D. W., and Chadwick, V. S.: Malabsorption and macroamylasemia. Amer. J. Med. 69: 451, 1980.
188. Höfler, H.: Symmetrische hämorrhagische Infarcierung der Ureteren als Komplikation der akuten Pankreatitis. Virchows Arch. Path. Anat. u. Histol. 379: 151, 1978.
189. Hoefler, H.: Pankreasnekrose. Todesursache, Überlebenszeit und Wahl des Operationszeitpunktes. Dtsch. med. Wschr. 104: 315, 1979.
190. Hoferichter, J.: Gezielte Prophylaxe der postoperativen Pankreasnekrose. Chirurg 78: 233, 1967.

191. Hollenberg, M., Kobold, E. E., Pruett, R., and Thal, A. P.: Occurrence of circulating vasoactive substances in human and experimental pancreatitis. Surg. Forum 13: 302, 1962.

192. Hollender, L. F.: Die dringliche Pankreatektomie bei der akuten Pankreatitis. Bericht über 17 eigene Beobachtungen. Langenbecks Arch. klin. Chir. 328: 314, 1971.

193. Hollender, L. F.: Chirurgie der akuten Pankreatitis. Langenbecks Arch. klin. Chir. 334: 337, 1973.

194. Hollender, L. F.: Le traitement chirurgical précoce des pancréatites aiguës. Chirurgie 100: 321, 1974.

195. Hollender, L. F.: Le traitement des pancréatites aiguës nécroticohémorragiques. Lyon Chirurgical 71: 91, 1975.

196. Hollender, L. F.: Traitement chirurgical de la pancréatite aiguë. Schweiz. med. Wschr. 106: 266, 1976.

197. Hollender, L. F.: Katastrophenherd Pankreas chirurgisch ausräumen. Ärztl. Praxis 30: 326, 1978.

198. Hollender, L. F.: Resection of the pancreas for acute hemorrhagic and necrotizing pancreatitis. World J. Surg. 3: 637, 1979.

199. Hollender, L. F.: Wann ist der Kallikreininhibitor in der Therapie der akuten Pankreatitis einzusetzen? Med. Welt 33: 1176, 1980.

200. Hollender, L. F.: Controversies in acute pancreatitis. Springer (Berlin), 1982.

201. Hollender, L. F., and Adloff, M.: Pancréatites aiguës nécrotico-hémorragiques. J. B. Bailliere et fils (Paris), 1963, p. 285.

202. Hollender, L. F., Gillet, M., and Otteni, F.: Pancréatite aiguë avec rupture du canal de Wirsung en péritoine libre. Mem. Acad. Chir. 97: 162, 1971.

203. Hollender, L. F., Gillet, M., and Sava, G.: La pancréatectomie d'urgence dans les pancréatites aiguës. A propos de 13 observations. Ann. Chir. 24: 647, 1970.

204. Hollender, L. F., Gillet, M., Sava, G., and Staub, D.: Les pancréatites aiguës postopératoires. Etude clinique et plaidoyer en faveur d'une réintervention plus systématique avec pancréatectomie précoce. J. Chir. 97: 177, 1969.

205. Hollender, L. F., Kohler, J. J., and Klein, A.: Zur chirurgischen Behandlung der akuten nekrotischen Pankreatitis. Chirurg 43: 256, 1972.

206. Hollender, L. F., Kohler, J. J., Klein, A., and Gillet, M.: A propos du traitement de la pancréatite aiguë nécrotico-hémorragique. Ann. Chir. 26: 649, 1972.

207. Hollender, L. F., Kohler, J. J., Weill, J. P., Dreyfus, J., and Winisdoerfer, G.: Les pancréatites aiguës gravidiques du postpartum. Ann. Chir. 26: 633, 1972.

208. Hollender, L. F., Kümmerle, F., Longmire, W. P., and Trede, M.: Chirurgie der Pankreatitis. Diskussionsforum. Langenbecks Arch. Chir. 338: 91, 1975.

209. Hollender, L. F., and Marrie, A.: Pseudozysten der Pankreas. In: M. Allgöwer et al. (Eds.): Chirurgische Gastroenterologie, Vol. 2. Springer (Berlin–Heidelberg–New York), 1981.

210. Hollender, L. F., and Marrie, A.: Nécroses pancréatiques. Encycl. Méd. Chir. Paris: Techniques chirurgicales. Appareil digestif, 40: 855.

211. Hollender, L. F., and Meyer, Ch.: A propos du procès verbal sur le traitement chirurgical des pancréatites aiguës. Chirurgie 103: 84, 1977.

212. Hollender, L. F., Meyer, Ch., Marrie, A., Da Silva e Costa, J. M., and Castellanos, J. G.: Role of surgery in the management of acute pancreatitis. World J. Surg. 5: 361: 1981.

213. Hollender, L. F., Meyer, Ch., Marrie, A., and Keller, D.: Etat actuel du traitement des pancréatites aiguës nécrotico-hémorragiques. J. Méd. Strasbourg 12: 329, 1981.

214. Hollender, L. F., Meyer, Ch., Marrie, A., and Keller, D.: Aktuelle Behandlung der nekrotisierend-hämorrhagischen Pankreatitis. Schwerpunkt Med. 1981, No. 3: Pankreas-Erkrankungen.

215. Hollender, L. F., Meyer, Ch., Otteni, F., and Dufour, A.: L'allergie aux antienzymes. Lyon Chir. 68: 200, 1972.

216. Hollender, L. F., Starlinger, M., and Meyer, Ch.: Die Chirurgie der akuten Pankreatitis. Akt. Chir. 12: 43, 1977.

217. Hollender, L. F., Viville, Ch., and Weiss, A. G.: Quelques réflexions à propos des biopsies pancréatiques. Lyon Chir. 60: 230, 1964.

218. Hollender, L. F., Viville, Ch., Schvingt, E., and Adloff, M.: Les lésions traumatiques du pancréas. Etude clinique et indications thérapeutiques. Arch. Mal. Appar. Dig. 51: 649, 1962.

219. Hotz, J.: Therapie der akuten Pankreatitis. Fortschr. Med. 94: 1193, 1976.

220. Hotz, J.: Akute Pankreatitis – neue Aspekte der konservativen Behandlung. Notfallmedizin 8: 57, 1982.

221. Hotz, J., and Goebell, H.: Ätiologie der akuten Pankreatitis. In: H. Sarles and M. Singer (Eds.): Akute und chronische Pankreatitis, p. 11. Witzstrock (Baden-Baden, Cologne, New York), 1978.

222. Howard, J. M.: Surgical diseases of the pancreas. Pitman (London), 1961.

223. Howard, J. M., and Jordan, G. L.: Relapsing pancreatitis secondary to choledocholithiasis. AMA Arch. Surg. 73: 960, 1956.

224. Howat, H. T., and Braganza, J. M.: Assessment of pancreatic dysfunction in man. In: H. T. Howat and H. Sarles (Eds.): The exocrine pancreas. Saunders (London–Philadelphia–Toronto), 1979.

225. Howes, R., Zuidema, G. D., and Cameron, J. L.: Evaluation of prophylactic antibiotics in acute pancreatitis. J. Surg. Res. 18: 197, 1975.

226. Hranilovich, G. D., and Beckenstoss, A. H.: Lesions of the pancreas in malignant hypertension. Arch. Path. 55: 443, 1953.

227. Imrie, C. W.: Pathophysiology of acute pancreatitis. Invited commentary. World J. Surg. 5: 323, 1981.

228. Imrie, C. W., Allam, B. F., and Ferguson, J. C.: Hypocalcaemia of acute pancreatitis: The effect of hypoalbuminaemia. Curr. Med. Res. Opin. 4: 101, 1976.

229. Imrie, C. W., Benjamin, I. S., Ferguson, J. C., McKay, A. J., Mackenzie, I., O'Neill, J., and Blumgart, L. H.: A single-centre double-blind trial of Trasylol therapy in primary acute pancreatitis. Brit. J. Surg. 65: 337, 1978.

230. Imrie, C. W., and Mackenzie, M.: Effective aprotinin therapie in canine experimental pancreatitis. Digestion 22: 32, 1981.

231. Jacobs, M. L., Daggett, W. M., and Civetta, J. M.: Acute pancreatitis: Analysis of factors influencing survival. Ann. Surg. 185: 43, 1977.

232. Jacobson, G., Hedstrand, U., and Nilson, B.: The cause of hypophosphatemia in acute pancreatitis. In: L. F. Hollender (Ed.): Constroversies in acute pancreatitis. Springer (Berlin–Heidelberg–New York), 1982.

233. Jalovaara, P.: Pancreatic exocrine secretion in the rat after chronic alcohol ingestion: Non-parallel secretion of proteins and pancreatic secretory trypsin inhibitor. Scand. J. Gastroent. 14: 57, 1979.

234. Jalovaara, P., and Apaja, M.: Alcohol and acute pancreatitis. An experimental study in the rat. Scand. J. Gastroent. 13: 703, 1978.

235. Johnson, H. L., Beaven, M. A., Erjavec, F., and Brodie, B. B.: Selective labelling and release of non-mast cell histamine. Life Sci. 5: 115, 1966.

236. Johnson, D. H., and Cornish, A. K.: Acute pancreatitis in patients receiving chlorothiazide. JAMA 170: 2054, 1959.

237. Jones, R. C., and Shires, G. T.: Pancreatic trauma. Arch. Surg. 102: 424, 1971.

238. Kasper, H., and Sommer, H.: Klinik der akuten Pankreatitis. In: M. Forell (Ed.): Handbuch der inneren Medizin, Vol. 3/6, 5th ed. Springer (Berlin–Heidelberg–New York), 1976.

239. Kast, A.: Bauchspeicheldrüse einschliesslich Inselorgan. In: E. Joest J. Dobberstein, G. Pallaske and H. Stürze (Eds.): Handbuch der speziellen pathologischen Anatomie der Haustiere, Vol. VI/2, 3rd ed. Parey (Berlin), 1967.

240. Kast, A., and Kersten, W.: Initialstadien einer akuten hämorrhagischen Pankreasnekrose beim Schwein. Berl. Münch. tierärztl. Wschr. 73: 336, 1960.

241. Kattwinkel, J. Lapey, A., and Di Sant'Agnese, P. A.: Hereditary pancreatitis: Three new kindreds and a critical review of the literature. Pediatrics 51: 55, 1973.

242. Keller, R.: Die Bedeutung der Gewebsmastzellen für die Entzündung. In: R. Heister and H. F. Hofmann (Eds.): Die Entzündung. Grundlagen und pharmakologische Beeinflussung, p. 132. Urban & Schwarzenberg (Munich–Berlin–Vienna), 1966.

243. Kelley, M. L.: A grey turner sigma not associated with acute pancreatitis. Gastroenterology 32: 142, 1957.

244. Kellum, J. M., Demeester, T. R., and Elskins, R. G.: Respiratory insufficiency secondary to acute pancreatitis. Ann. Surg. 175: 657, 1972.

245. Kelly, T. R.: Gallstone pancreatitis pathophysiology. Surgery 80: 488, 1976.

246. Kelly, A. G., and Nahrwold, D. L.: Pancreatic secretion in response to an elemental diet and intravenous hyperalimentation. Surg. Gynec. Obstet. 143: 87, 1976.

247. Kimura, T., Toung, S. K., and Margolis, S.: Respiratory failure in acute pancreatitis. Ann. Surg. 189: 509, 1979.

248. Kivilakso, E., Fräki, O., Nikki, P., and Lempinen, M.: Resection of the pancreas for acute fulminant pancreatitis. Surg. Gynec. Obstet. 152: 493, 1981.

249: Klatskin, G., and Gordon, M.: Relationship between relapsing pancreatitis and essential hyperlipemia. Amer. J. Med. 12: 3, 1952.

250. Klemm, G., Putzke, H.-P., and Rohde, L.: Urethannarkose und Pankreasschaden. Dtsch. Z. Verdau. Stoffwechselkr. 31: 123, 1972.

251. Klose, G., Klapdor, R., and Greten, H.: Akute Pankreatitis: Stoffwechselveränderungen sind diagnostische and prognostische Parameter. Klinikarzt 11: 616, 1982.

252. Korb, G., Müller, R., Gedigk, P., and Helwig, K.: Über die Entstehung und Abheilung von Lebernekrosen nach einem einmaligen Schock. Virchows Arch., Abt. A 348: 374, 1969.

253. Korn, K. J.: Hämorrhagisch-nekrotisierende Pankreatitis durch lokales Shwartzman-Phänomen. Ihre Abgrenzung von der tryptischen Pankreatitis. Frankfurt. Z. Path. 73: 203, 1963.

254. Kössling, F. K., Nagel, M., and Schäfer, A.: Experimentelle tryptische Pankreatitis durch metabolische Läsion. Serologische, histologische und elektronenmikroskopische Untersuchungen. Z. Gastroent. 5: 185, 1967.

255. Kraus, S.: Endoscopic sphincterotomy – An emergency intervention in acute biliary-type pancreatitis. Endoscopy U. 283, 1979.

256. Kronborg, O., Bülow, S., Joergensen, P. M., and Svendsen, L. B.: A randomized double-blind trial of glucagon in treatment of first attack of severe acute pancreatitis without associated biliary disease. Amer. J. Gastroent. 73: 423, 1980.

257. Kümmerle, F.: Frühindikation der akuten Pankreatitis: Operation. Langenbecks Arch. Chir., Kongressbericht, p. 563, 1978.

258. Kümmerle, F., Neher, M., Schönborn, H., and Mangold, G.: Vorzeitige Operation bei akuter hämorrhagisch-nekrotisierender Pankreatitis. Dtsch. med. Wschr. 100: 2241, 1975.

259. Kümmerle, F., and Schönborn, H.: Possibilities and limits of intensive care in acute necrotic pancreatitis. International Symposium, Strasbourg, June 12–13, 1981: Controversies in acute pancreatitis.

260. Kune, G. A.: The challenge of severe acute pancreatitis. Med. J. Aust. 2: 8, 1968.

261. Lackner, K., Frommhold, H., Grauthoff, H., Mödder, U., Heuser, L., Braun, G., Buurman, R., and Scherer, K.: Wertigkeit der Computertomographie und der Sonographie innerhalb der Pankreasdiagnostik. Fortschr. Röntgenstr. 132: 509, 1980.

262. Lagache, G., and Vankemmel, M.: Modalités du traitement lésionnel des pancréatites aiguës nécrosantes. Mém. Acad. Chir. 100: 394, 1974.

263. Lagache, G., Vankemmel, M., Edelmann, G., Boutelier, P., Guivarc'H, M., Hollender, L. F., Colin, R., and Bories-Azeau, A.: Le traitement des pancréatites aiguës nécrosantes par l'ablation chirurgicale précoce des portions nécrosées. Chirurgie 100: 155, 1974.

264. Lake-Bakaar, G., McKavanagh, S., Gatus, B., and Summerfield, J. A.: The relative values of serum immunoactive trypsin concentration and total amylase activity in the diagnosis of mumps, chronic renal failure, and pancreatic disease. Scand. J. Gastroent. 15: 97, 1980.

265. Langer, S., and Zilkens, K. W.: Postoperative Pankreatitis nach Oberbaucheingriffen. In: Aktuelle Chirurgie: Die Chirurgie der akuten und chronischen Pankreatitis. TM-Verlag 1980, Symposion Berlin (R. Häring, Ed.).

266. Lankisch, P. G.: Therapie der akuten Pankreatitis: Tierexperimentelle Untersuchungen. Thieme (Stuttgart), 1980.

267. Lankisch, P. G.: Laparoskopie bei akuter Pankreatitis? Dtsch. med. Wschr. 107: 755, 1982.

268. Lankisch, P. G.: Konservative Therapie der akuten Pankreatitis. Dtsch. med. Wschr. 107: 630, 1982.

269. Lankisch, P. G., and Creutzfeldt, W.: Akute und akut rezidivierende Pankreatitis. In: M. Allgöwer, F. Harder, L. F. Hollender, H. J. Peiper, and J. R. Siewert (Eds.): Chirurgische Gastroenterologie, Vol. 2. Springer (Berlin–Heidelberg–New York), 1981.

270. Lankisch, P. G., Göke, B., Kunze, H., Otto, J., Winckler, K., and Creutzfeldt, W.: Has PGE_2 a protective effect in pancreatitis? Digestion 25: 48, 1982 b.

271. Lankisch, P. G., Koop, H., and Winckler, K.: Continuous peritoneal dialysis treatment of acute experimental pancreatitis in the rat: I. Effect on length and rate of survival. Dig. Dis. Sci. 24: 111, 1979.

272. Lankisch, P. G., Koop, H., and Winckler, K.: Continuous peritoneal dialysis treatment of acute experimental pancreatitis in the rat: II. Analysis of its beneficial effect. Dig. Dis. Sci. 24: 117, 1979.

References

273. Lankisch, P. G., Koop, H., Otto, J., and Oberdieck, U.: Evaluation of methaemalbumin in acute pancreatitis. Scand. J. Gastroent. 13: 975, 1978.
274. Lankisch, P. G., Koop, H., Winckler, K., Fölsch, U. R., and Creutzfeldt, W.: Somatostatin therapy of acute experimental pancreatitis. Gut 18: 713, 1977.
275. Lankisch, P. G., Lopez, E., Winckler, K., and Schuster, R.: Kolonveränderungen nach Pankreatitis. Dtsch. med. Wschr. 101: 1885, 1976.
276. Lataste, J., and Serpault, P.: Le traitement chirurgical des pancréatites aiguës hémorragiques. J. Chir. 113: 447, 1977.
277. Lawson, D. W., Daggett, W. M., Civetta, J. M., Corry, R. H., and Bartlett, M. K.: Surgical treatment of acute necrotizing pancreatitis. Ann. Surg. 172: 605, 1970.
278. Leborgne, J., Pannier, M., Le Neel, J. C., Potiron, L., and Visset, J.: Lésions coliques au cours des pancréatites nécrosantes. A propos de 4 observations. Ann. Chir. 30: 377, 1976.
279. Leger, L., Chiche, B., and Ghouti, A.: Notre expérience de la pancréatite aiguë. Chirurgie 103: 846, 1977.
280. Leger, L., Chiche, B., Moulle, P., and Louvel, A.: Pancreatic necrosis and acute pancreatitis. Int. Surg. 63: 41, 1979.
281. Leger, L., Liguory, C., Coffin, J. Ch., Chiche, B., and Desfemmes, F.: La sphincterotomie endoscopique dans la pancréatite aiguë. Chirurgie 105: 772, 1979.
282. Leger, L., Parc, R., and Soprani, A.: Chronic familial pancreatitis: 13 cases, five families. J. Chir. 115: 129, 1978.
283. Lehnert, P.: Ätiologie und Pathogenese der chronischen Pankreatitis. Internist 20: 321, 1979.
284. Lemoine, G. H., and Lapasset, F.: Un cas de pancréatite ourlienne avec autopsie. Bull. Mém. Soc. Hôp. Paris 22: 640, 1905.
285. Levant, J. A., Secrist, D. M., Resin, H., Sturdevant, R. A. L., and Guth, P. H.: Nasogastric suction in the treatment of alcoholic pancreatitis. JAMA 229: 51, 1974.
286. Levy, A.: Association infarctus du myocarde et pancréatite aiguë. Presse méd. 73: 1345, 1965; Ann. Chir. 19: 171, 1965.
287. Lilja, P., Evander, A., and Ihse, I.: Hereditary pancreatitis: A report on two kindreds. Acta Chir. Scand. 144: 35, 1978.
288. Limberg, B., and Kommerell, B.: Treatment of acute pancreatitis with somatostatin. New Eng. J. Med. 303: 284, 1980.
289. Lindner, H.: Akute Pankreatitis (Pankreasnekrose) infolge Glucocorticoidtherapie. Dtsch. med. Wschr. 89: 833, 1964.
290. Link, M.: Sektionsbefunde bei postoperativer Pankreasnekrose. Zbl. Chir. 90: 2211, 1965.
291. Löffler, A., Löffler-Bock, A. H., and Friedrichs, U.: Hyperlipoproteinämie und Pankreatitis. Leber, Magen, Darm 6: 249, 1976.
292. Lorentz, K.: Untersuchungen zur klinischen Wertigkeit der Lipase- und α-Amylasebestimmung im Serum bei Pankreatitis. Z. Gastroent. 18: 543, 1980.
293. Ludlow, A. I.: Autopsy incidence of cholelithiasis. Amer. J. Med. Sci. 193: 481, 1937.
294. Lutz, H., and Ehler, R.: Ultraschalldiagnostik des Pankreas. Therapiewoche 28: 6900, 1978.
295. Malik, S. A., van Kley, H., and Knight, W. A.: Inherited defect in hereditary pancreatitis. Dig. Dis. Sci. 22: 999, 1977.
296. Mallet-Guy, P., and Feroldi, J.: Bases pathologiques expérimentales et cliniques de la splanchnicectomie gauche dans le traitement des pancréatites chroniques recidivantes. Presse méd. 99, 1953.
297. Mallet-Guy, P., Feroldi, J., and Reboul, E.: Recherches expérimentales sur la pathogénie des pancréatites aiguës. Leur provocation par l'excitation du nerf splanchnique gauche. Lyon Chir. 44: 281, 1949.
298. Mallet-Guy, P., and Giura, F.: Reflux Wirsungien et pancréatites. Analyse d'une deuxième série de 400 cas de reflux cholangiographique dans le canal de Wirsung. Lyon Chir. 53: 481, 1957.
299. Mallet-Guy, P., Jeanjean, R., and Feroldi, J.: Provocation expérimentale de pancréatites aiguës par excitation électrique du splanchnique gauche. Lyon Chir. 39: 437, 1944.
300. Mallory, A., and Kern, F., Jr.: Drug-induced pancreatitis. A critical review. Gastroent. 78: 813, 1980.
301. Manabe, T., and Steer, M. L.: Protease inhibitors and experimental acute hemorrhagic pancreatitis. Ann. Surg. 190: 13, 1979.
302. Manegold, B. C.: Diagnostische und operative Endoskopie im oberen Ga-

strointestinaltrakt. In: Breitner: Operationslehre 1, Beitrag 9, 1982.

303. Marks, I. N., Bank, S., and Barbezat, G. O.: Alkoholpankreatitis – Ätiologie, klinische Formen, Komplikationen. Leber, Magen, Darm 6: 257: 1976.

304. Maroske, D., Thon, K., and Röher, H. D.: Haemorrhagisch-nekrotisierende Pankreatitis: Beeinflussung der Operationsindikation durch die therapeutische Peritoneallavage. Private communication, 1982.

305. Martin, D. M., Someren, A. O., and Nasrallah, S. M.: The effect of prostaglandin E_2 on ethionine-induced pancreatitis in the rat. Gastroenterology 81: 736, 1981.

306. Mashoff, W., Lindlar, F., and Stolpmann, H. J.: Morphologische und lipidchemische Untersuchungen zur Autolyse von Leber und Pankreas. Virchows Arch. path. Anat. 337: 340, 1964.

307. May, B., Holler, C., and Westmann, E.: Über die Bedeutung der Phospholipase A für die histaminfreisetzende Wirkung des Cobragiftes. Naunyn-Schmiedebergs Arch. exp. Path. Pharmak. 256: 237, 1967.

308. McCarthy, M. C., and Dickermann, M. R.: Surgical management of severe acute pancreatitis. Arch. Surg. 117: 476, 1982.

309. McCutcheon, A.: A fresh approach to the pathogenesis of pancreatitis. Gut 9: 296, 1968.

310. McMahon, M. J.: Peritoneal lavage for the diagnosis and prognosis of acute pancreatitis. In: L. F. Hollender (Ed.): Controversies in acute pancreatitis. Springer (Berlin–Heidelberg–NewYork), 1982.

311. McMahon, M. J., Playforth, M. J., and Pickford, I. R.: A comparative study of methods of the prediction of severity of attacks of acute pancreatitis. Brit. J. Surg. 67: 22, 1980.

312. Medical Research Council Multicentre Trial: Morbidity of acute pancreatitis: The effect of aprotinin and glucagon. Gut 21: 334, 1980.

313. Menguy, R. B., Hallenbeck, G. H., Bollmann, J. L., and Grindlay, J. H.: Intraductal pressures and sphincteric resistance in canine pancreatic and biliary ducts after various stimuli. S.G.O. 106: 306, 1958.

314. Mercadier, M.: Sur une série de 100 cas de pancréatites aiguës graves opérés précocement. Chirurgie 103: 835, 1977.

315. Mercadier, M., and Chigot, J. P.: Indications and surgical methods in severe acute necrotic pancreatitis. International Symposium Strasbourg, June 12–13, 1981. Controversies in acute pancreatitis.

316. Meyer, Ch., Otteni, F., and Hollender, L. F.: A propos d'un cas d'allergie aux inhibiteurs de protéases. Presse méd. 79: 2495, 1971.

317. Millbourn, E.: On the excretory ducts of the pancreas in man with special reference to their relations to each other, to the common bile duct and to the duodenum. A radiological and anatomical study. Acta anat. (Basle) 9: 1, 1950.

318. Miller, J. M.: Trasylol in primary acute pancreatitis. Brit. J. Surg. 65: 887, 1978.

319. Molander, D. W., and Bell, E. T.: Relation of cholelithiasis to acute pancreatitis. A.M.A. Arch. Path. 41: 17, 1946.

320. Mölbert, E.: Die Orthologie und Pathologie der Zelle im elektronenmikroskopischen Bild. In: Handbuch der allgemeinen Pathologie, Vol. II/5, p. 238. Springer (Berlin–Heidelberg–New York), 1968.

321. Molnar, J. J., Schneider, I. J., Tindel, S., Shapira, D., and State, D.: Hemorrhagic pancreatitis induced by elastase. Acta Morph. Acad. Sci. Hung. 16: 213, 1968.

322. Morris, R. E.: Studies on the development of pancreatic necrosis in the living mouse. Bull. Johns Hopkins Hosp. 114: 212, 1964.

323. Mouiel, J.: Rôle de la millilithiase biliaire dans la pathogénie des pancréatites aiguës. Nouv. Presse Méd. 11: 1855, 1982.

324. Mouiel, J., Chauvin, P., Borelli, J. P., Bus, J. J., Giaume, F., and Bourgeon, R.: Le rôle de la microlithiase biliaire dans les pancréatites aiguës. Chirurgie 101: 258, 1975.

325. Mullen, J. L., Buzby, G. P., Matthews, D. C., Smale, B. F., and Rosato, E. F.: Reduction of operative morbidity and mortality by combined preoperative and postoperative nutritional support. Ann. Surg. 192: 604, 1980.

326. Multinger, L., Figarella, C., and Sarles, H.: Diagnosis of chronic pancreatitis by measurement of lactoferrin in duodenal juice. Gut 22: 350, 1981.

327. Nagel, M.: Tierexperimentelle und klinische Untersuchungen zur zusätzlichen Therapie mit Proteasen-Inhibitoren bei der Perforationsperitonitis. Bull. Soc. Int. Chir. 27: 214, 1968.

328. Nagel, M.: Trasylol und Peritonitis. Langenbecks Arch. klin. Chir. (Kongressband 325): 327, 1969.

329. Nagel, M.: Metablisch bedingte Pankreatitis. Giessen Pancreas Symposium 1967. Schattauer (Stuttgart), 1969.

330. Nagel, M.: Aktuelle Aspekte der Pankreatitis-Chirurgie. Chirurg 43: 241, 1972.

331. Nagel, M.: Maligner und benigner Verschluss-Ikterus. Langenbecks Arch. klin. Chir. 327: 496, 1970.

332. Nagel, M.: Zur Frage der Schmerzbeeinflussung bei der chronischen Pankreatitis durch Proteasen-Inhibitor-Therapie und Operation. Int. Symposium: Clinical Enzyme Inhibitor Therapy, Strasbourg, 1970.

333. Nagel, M.: Spezielle pathophysiologische Aspekte bei akuter und chronischer Pankreatitis. Langenbecks Arch. klin. Chir. 334: 351, 1973.

334. Nagel, M.: Indikationen für die Chirurgie der akuten Pankreatitis Pancreas Symposium, Surgical University Clinic, Hamburg, 1975.

335. Nagel, M.: Das Pankreas als Reaktionsorgan bei Herz- und Kreislauferkrankungen. In: M. M. Forell (Ed.): Handbuch der inneren Medizin, Vol. 3/6. Springer (Berlin–Heidelberg), 1976.

336. Nagel, M., Junghanns, K., and Encke, A.: Das stumpfe und penetrierende Bauchtrauma. In: Chirurgie der Gegenwart, Vol. IVa. Urban & Schwarzenberg (Munich), 1976.

337. Nagel, W., Robel, K. P., and Willig, F.: Über die Aktivierung proteolytischer Proenzyme des Pankreas. Klin. Wschr. 43: 173, 1965.

338. Nager, F., and Steiner, H.: Der Pankreasinfarkt bei maligner Hypertonie. Schweiz. med. Wschr. 95: 119, 1965.

339. Neher, M., Braun, B., and Klose, K. J.: Der Einfluss von Sonographie und Computertomographie auf die operative Behandlung der akuten Pankreatitis. Langenbecks Arch. klin. Chir. 356: 141, 1982.

340. Neher, M., and Kümmerle, F.: Gastrointestinale Komplikationen bei akuter Pankreatitis. Dtsch. med. Wschr. 103: 1400, 1978.

341. Neumayr, A., and Peschl, L.: Zusammenhänge zwischen Gallenblasen- und Pankreaserkrankungen. In: W. Boecker (Ed.): Gallenblase, Pankreas. Thieme (Stuttgart), 1975.

342. Neurath, H.: Consideration of the occurrence, structure and function of the proteolytic enzymes of the pancreas. In: Ciba Foundation Symposium on the exocrine pancreas. Churchill (London), 1961.

343. Nevalainen, T. J.: The role of phospholipase A in acute pancreatitis. Scand. J. Gastroent. 15: 641, 1980.

344. Noore, W. R., Canton, H. H., and Raines, D. R.: Peritoneal lavage in the treatment of acute pancreatitis ascites. Am. J. Gastroenterol. 69: 88, 1978.

345. Norton, L., and Eiseman, B.: Near total pancreatectomy for hemorrhagic pancreatitis. Amer. J. Surg. 127: 191, 1974.

346. Novis, I. M.: Partial obstruction of the pancreatic duct by round worms, Brit. J. Surg. 10: 421, 1923.

347. Nugent, F. W., Bulan, M. B., and Zuberi, S.: Intraarterial antienzymes in experimental pancreatitis. Clin. Res. 16: 289, 1968.

348. Nugent, F. W., Zuberi, S., and Bulan, M. B.: Kinin precursor in experimental pancreatitis. Proc. Soc. Exp. Biol. 130: 566, 1969.

349. Öfler, H.: Pankreasnekrose, Todesursachen, Überlebenszeit und Wahl des Operationszeitpunktes. Dtsch. med. Wschr. 104: 315, 1979.

350. Ohlsson, K., and Eddeland, A.: Release of proteolytic enzymes in bileinduced pancreatitis in dogs. Gastroenterology 69: 668, 1975.

351. Olazabal, A., and Nascimento, L.: Effects of indomethacin, aspirin and fat-free diet on experimental pancreatitis in the rat. J. Lab. Clin. Med. 96: 570, 1980.

352. Olivero de Rubiana, J. P., Duron, J. J., Barbe, D., Validire, J., and Viars, P.: Alimentation entérale précoce par cathéter jéjunal en chirurgie digestive lourde. Nouv. Presse Méd. 11: 447, 1982.

353. Olson, T.: Lipomatosis of the pancreas in autopsy material and its relation to age and overweight. Acta Path. Microbil. Scand., Sect. A, 86: 367.

354. Otte, M.: Pankreasfunktionsdiagnostik. Internist 20: 331, 1979.

355. Palielo, L. G., and Gallanger, H. S.: Anomalous termination of pancreatic duct. Report of case with chronic biliary obstruction. Arch. Path. (Chicago) 71: 381, 1961.

356. Papp, M. D.: About the acinar-enzymatic, vascular-inflammatory and interstial-lymphatic components in the origin of acute pancreas necrosis. Thesis, University of Budapest, 1970.

357. Papp, M. D., Fodor, J., and Makara, G. B.: Bradykinin-induced histological

changes in the pancreas. Z. ges. exp. Med. 147: 264, 1968.

358. Papp, M. D., Nemeth, P., and Horvath, E. J.: Pancreatico-duodenal lymph flow and lipase activity in acute experimental pancreatitis. Lymphology 4: 48, 1971.

359. Paul, F., Ohnhaus, E. E., Hesch, R. D., Chemnitz, G., Hoppe-Seyler, R., Henrichs, H. R., Hartung, H., Waldmann, D., Kunze, K., Barth, E., Nüesch, E., and Abt, K.: Einfluss von Salm-Calcitonin auf den Verlauf der akuten Pankreatitis. Dtsch. med. Wschr. 104: 615, 1979.

360. Pham Bieu Tam: Pancréatite aiguë due à la présence d'ascaris dans la voie biliaire principale. West. J.S.G.O. 67: 270, 1959.

361. Pichlmaier, H., and Junginger, T.: Kommentar zur "Diagnostik und Therapie der akuten Pankreatitis" (c. o.). Leber, Magen, Darm 10: 12, 1980.

362. Pizzecco, E.: Akute Pankreatitis und Pankreatose. Münch. med. Wschr. 102: 795, 1960.

363. Pringot, J., Dardenne, A. N., Lousse, J. P., Reynaert, M., and Kestens, P. J.: Contribution of computer tomography in the diagnosis of severe acute pancreatitis. Int. Symposium Strasbourg, June 12–13, 1981: Controversies in acute pancreatitis.

364. Probstein, J. G.: Acute pancreatitis. J. Inter. Coll. Surg. 15: 147, 1951.

365. Probstein, J. G., and Sachar, L. A.: Acute pancreatitis: Questions and answers. Surg. Clin. N. Amer. 30: 1457, 1950.

366. Rahlf, G., Lankisch, P. G., Koop, H., and Cöll, H. B.: Lungenveränderungen bei akuter haemorrhagischer Pankreatitis. Verh. dtsch. Ges. Path. 63: 545.

367. Raithel, D., and Mühe, E.: Akute Pankreatitis nach Operation mittels extrakorporaler Zirkulation. Chirurg 41: 518, 1970.

368. Ranson, J. H. C.: Surgical treatment of acute pancreatitis. Dig. Dis. Sci. 25: 453, 1980.

369. Ranson, J. H. C.: Conservative surgical treatment of acute pancreatitis. World J. Surg. 5: 351, 1981.

370. Ranson, J. H. C.: The timing of biliary surgery in acute pancreatitis. Ann. Surg. 189: 654.

371. Ranson, J. H. C., Facs, B. M. B., and Pasternack, B. S.: Statistical method for quantifying the severity of clinical acute pancreatitis. J. Surg. Res. 22: 79, 1977.

372. Ranson, J. H. C., Rifkind, K. M., Roses, D. F., Fink, S. D., Eng, K., and Spencer, F. C.: Prognostic signs and the role of operative management in acute pancreatitis. Surg. Gyn. Obstet. 139: 69, 1974.

373. Ranson, J. H. C., Rifkind, K. M., and Turner, J. W.: Prognostic signs and nonoperative peritoneal lavage in acute pancreatitis. Surg. Gyn. Obstet. 143: 209, 1976.

374. Ranson, J. H. C., and Spencer, F. C.: The role of peritoneal lavage in severe acute pancreatitis. Ann. Surg. 187: 565, 1978.

375. Ranson, J. H. C., Turner, B. J. W., Roses, D. F., Rifkind, K. M., and Spencer, F. C.: Respiratory complications in acute pancreatitis. Ann. Surg. 179: 557, 1974.

376. Rao, N. K., Zuretti, M. F., Maccino, F. M., and Lombardi, B.: Acute hemorrhagic pancreatic necrosis in mice. The activity of lysosomal enzymes in the pancreas and the liver. Amer. J. Path. 98: 45, 1980.

377. Regan, P. T., Malagelada, J.-R., Go, V. L. W., Wolf, A. M., and DiMagno, E. P.: A prospective study of the antisecretory and therapeutic effects of cimetidine and glucagon in human acute pancreatitis. Mayo Clin. Proc. 56: 499, 1981.

378. Reid, B. G., and Kune, G. A.: Accuracy in diagnosis of acute pancreatitis. Med. J. Aust. 1: 583, 1978.

379. Reming, Y. H., Priestly, J. T., Judd, E. S., and King, J. N.: Total pancreatectomy. Ann. Surg. 172: 595, 1970.

380. Riccardi, V. M., Shih, V. E., and Holmes, L. B.: Hereditary pancreatitis: Nonspecificity of aminoaciduria and diagnosis of occult disease. Arch. Intern. Med. 135: 822, 1975.

381. Rick, W.: Messung von Enzymaktivitäten. In: M. M. Forell (Ed.): Handbuch der inneren Medizin, 5th ed., Vol. 3/6. Springer (Berlin–Heidelberg–New York), 1976.

382. Rigby, H. M.: Acute hemorrhagic pancreatitis, round worm in pancreatic duct. Brit. J. Surg. 10: 419, 1923.

383. Riley, J. F.: Mast cells and cancer in the skin of mice. Lancet, p. 1457, 1966.

384. Ritter, U.: Erkrankungen des exkretorischen Pankreas. Thieme (Stuttgart), 1971.

385. Roberts, N. J., Baggenstoss, A. H., and Comfort, M. W.: Acute pancreatic necrosis. A clinicopathological study. Amer. J. Clin. Pathol. 20: 742, 1950.

386. Robinson, A. S.: Acute pancreatitis following translumbar aortography. Arch. Surg. 2: 72, 1956.

387. Rodgers, R. E., and Carey, L. C.: Peritoneal lavage in experimental pancreatitis in dogs. Am. J. Surg. 111: 792, 1966.

388. Rosato, E. F., Mullis, W. F., and Rosato, F. E.: Peritoneal lavage therapy in hemorrhagic pancreatitis. Surgery 74: 106, 1973.

389. Rosenberg, V., and Dreiling, D. A.: The effect of prolactin on canine pancreatic secretion. Implications on the pathogenesis of the pancreatitis pregnancy. Am. J. Gastroenterol. 67: 354, 1977.

390. Ryan, J. W., Moffat, J. G., and Thompson, A. C.: Role of bradykinin system in acute hemorrhagic pancreatitis. Arch. Surg. 91: 14, 1965.

391. Sabrazes, J.: Lombricose du canal de Wirsung: pancréatite aiguë hémorragique. Ann. Anat. Path. 2: 385, 1925.

392. Safrany, L.: Endoscopic sphincterotomy in acute gallstone-induced pancreatitis. Int. Symposium Strasbourg, June 12–13, 1981: Controversies in acute pancreatitis.

393. Safrany, L., Neuhaus, B., Krause, S., Portocarrero, G., and Schott, B.: Endoskopische Papillotomie bei akuter, biliär bedingter Pankreatitis. Dtsch. med. Wschr. 105: 115, 1980.

394. Safrany, L., and Schott, B.: Endoskopische Papillotomie bei akuter biliärer Pankreatitis. In: H. Bartelheimer, F.-W. Ossenberg, and H. W. Schreiber (Eds.): Die kranken Gallenwege. Witzstrock (Baden-Baden, Cologne, New York), 1980.

395. Sandritter, W., and Lasch, H. G.: Pathologic aspects of shock. Meth. Achiev. Exp. Path. 3: 86, 1966.

396. Sarles, H.: An international survey on nutrition and pancreatitis. Digestion 9: 389, 1973.

397. Sarles, H.: Preface to Issue No. 4/76. Leber, Magen, Darm 6: 195, 1976.

398. Sarles, H.: Alcohol and the pancreas. Nutr. Metab. 21: 175, 1977.

399. Sarles, H., Sahel, J., Guien, C., Payan, H., and Sarles J.-C.: Die chronische Pankreatitis. In: M. M. Forell (Ed.): Handbuch der inneren Medizin, Vol. 3/6. Springer (Berlin–Heidelberg–New York), 1976.

400. Sarles, H., Sarles, J. C., Camatte, R., Muratore, R., Guien, M., Guien, C., Pastor, J., and Leroy, F.: Observations on 205 confirmed cases of acute pancreatitis, recurring pancreatitis and chronic pancreatitis. Gut 6: 545, 1965.

401. Sarles, H., Singer, M., and Sahel, J.: Pathologische Anatomie, Pathogenese und Ätiologie der chronischen Pankreatitis. In: H. Sarles and M. Singer (Eds.): Akute und chronische Pankreatitis. Witzstrock (Baden-Baden, Cologne, New York), 1978.

402. Sarles, H., Tiscornia, O., and Sahel, J.: Ätiologie und Pathogenese der chronischen Pankreatitis. Leber, Magen, Darm 6: 206, 1976b.

403. Satake, K., Rosmanith, J. S., and Appert, H. E.: Hypotension and release of kinin-forming enzyme into ascitic fluid exudate during experimental pancreatitis in dogs. Ann. Surg. 177: 497, 1973.

404. Scherer, U.: Computertomographische Untersuchungen der Oberbauchorgane. Internist 19: 579, 1978.

405. Schmidt, H.: Neuere Vorstellungen zur Pathogenese der akuten Pankreatitis. Internist 11: 105, 1970.

406. Schmidt, H.: Klinisch-diagnostische Gesichtspunkte und konservative Therapie der Pankreatitiden. Therapiewoche 27: 4961, 1977.

407. Schmidt, H., and Creutzfeldt, W.: The possible role of phospholipase A in the pathogenesis of acute pancreatitis. Scand. J. Gastroent. 4: 39, 1969.

408. Schmidt, H., Creutzfeldt, W., and Habermann, E.: Phospholipase A – ein möglicherweise entscheidender Faktor in der Pathogenese der akuten Pankreatitis. Klin. Wschr. 45: 163, 1967.

409. Schmidt, H., and Lankisch, P. G.: Fettgewebsnekrose, eine Ursache der pankreatischen Parenchymnekrose? Digestion 17: 84, 1978.

410. Schmitz-Moormann, P., and Böger, A.: Tissue damage by fatty acids released by lipolysis: Contribution to the pathogenesis of acute pancreatitis. Path. Res. Pract. 171: 303, 1981.

411. Schmitz-Moormann, P., and Keilos, E.: Morphologische Veränderungen bei der experimentellen temporären Ischämie des Katzenpankreas. Z. Gastroent. 9: 673, 1971.

412. Schönbach, G.: Änderungen der Mikrozirkulation bei der akuten Pankreatitis. In: Neue Aspekte der Trasylol-Therapie III. Schattauer (Stuttgart–New York), 1969.

413. Schönborn, H.: Intensivmedizin bei akuter Pankreatitis. Intensivmed. 10: 299, 1973.

414. Schönborn, H., and Kümmerle, F.: Die akute Pankreatitis und ihre Intensivtherapie. Intensivmed. 15: 39, 1978.

415. Schönborn, H., Kümmerle, F., Neher, M., and Schuster, H.-P.: Akute Pankreatitis. Entwicklung eines kombinierten konservativ-operativen Therapiekonzepts. Med. Welt 27: 1293, 1976.

416. Schönborn, H., Neher, M., and Kümmerle, F.: Kommentar zur "Diagnostik und Therapie der akuten Pankreatitis" (c.o.). Leber, Magen, Darm 10: 14, 1980.

417. Schönborn, H., Pross, E., and Olbermann, M.: Neuere Vorstellungen zur konservativen und operativen Therapie der akuten Pankreatitis. Internist 16: 108, 1975.

418. Schramm, W.: Private communication.

419. Schröder, T.: Phospholipase A_2 in acute pancreatitis. An experimental and clinical study. Heinonen Ky Nakkila, Helsinki, 1981.

420. Schröder, T., Kivilaakso, E., Kinnunen, P. K. J., and Lempinen, M.: Serum phospholipase A_2 in human acute pancreatitis. Scand. J. Gastroent. 15: 633, 1980.

421. Schröder, T., Lempinen, M., Nordling, S., and Kinnunen, P. K. J.: Chlorpromazine treatment of experimental acute fulminant pancreatitis in pigs. Eur. Surg. Res. 13: 143, 1981.

422. Schröder, T., Somerharju, P., and Lempinen, M.: Phospholipase A_2 in serum and ascitic exudate in experimental acute hemorrhagic pancreatitis in pigs. Eur. Surg. Res. 11: 172, 1979.

423. Schuster, H. P., Neher, M., Schönborn, H., and Kümmerle, F.: Akutes Nieren- und Lungenversagen bei diffuser Peritonitis und hämorrhagisch-nekrotisierender Pankreatitis. Dtsch. med. Wschr. 105: 82, 1980.

424. Schwedes, U., Althoff, P. H., Klempa, I., Leuschner, U., Mathes, L., Raptis, S., Wdowinski, J., and Usadel, K. H.: Effect of somatostatin on bile-induced acute hemorrhagic pancreatitis in the dog. Horm. Metab. Res. 11: 655, 1979.

425. Schwerk, W. B.: Ultraschalldiagnostik in der Gastroenterologie. Indikationen und Ergebnisse. Internist 23: 36, 1982.

426. Seelig, R., and Seelig, H. P.: Complement-mediated acinar cell necroses in pancreatitis induced by basement membrane antibodies. Virchows Arch. Abt. A 371: 69, 1976.

427. Seifert, G.: Zur Pathologie des kindlichen Pankreas bei akuten und chronischen Ernährungsstörungen. Beitr. path. Anat. 114: 1, 1954.

428. Seifert, G.: Die Pathologie des kindlichen Pankreas. Leipzig, 1956.

429. Seifert, G.: Zur Pathologie der Pankreatitis im Kindesalter. Mschr. Kinderheilk. 108: 225, 1960.

430. Seifert, G.: Mundhöhle, Mundspeicheldrüse, Tonsillen und Rachen. Spezielle pathologische Anatomie, Vol. 1. Springer (Berlin–Heidelberg–New York), 1966.

431. Seifert, G.: Das Pankreas als Schockorgan. In: K. Horatz (Ed.): Leber- und Pankreasschäden durch Schock und Narkose, p. 17. Thieme (Stuttgart), 1970.

432. Selby, J.: Acute pancreatitis; a review of present concepts as related to forty-six cases in the District of Columbia. M. Ann. (Columbia) 18: 671, 1949.

433. Selye, H.: The mast cells. Butterworths (London), 1965.

434. Shanklin, D. R.: Pancreatic atrophy apparently secondary to hydrochlorothiazide. New Eng. J. Med. 266: 1097, 1962.

435. Sibert, J. R.: A British family with hereditary pancreatitis. Gut 16: 81, 1975.

436. Siegel, M., and Werner, M.: Allergische Pankreatitis bei einer Sensibilisierung gegen den Kallikrein-Trupsin-Inaktivator. Dtsch. med. Wschr. 90: 1712, 1965.

437. Simon, G. T., and Giacobino, J. P.: Pathogenesis of the glomerular lesions in acute pancreatitis. Lancet II: 669, 1970.

438. Soergel, K. H.: Medical treatment of acute pancreatitis. Gastroenterology 74: 620, 1978.

439. Staudacher, V. and Martinotti, A.: Possibilità terapeutiche e di urgenza nelle pancreatitis acute. Minerva Chir. 31: 515, 1976.

440. Steinberg, D.: On leaving the peritoneal cavity open in acute generalized suppurative pancreatitis. Amer. J. Surg. 137: 216, 1979.

441. Steinberg, W. M., and Lewis, J. H.: Steroid-induced pancreatitis: Does it really exist? Gastroenterology 81: 799, 1981.

442. Stepanow, S.: Histologische und histochemische Veränderungen im exokrinen Pankreasgewebe bei Arteriosklerose und Hypertonie. Arch. Path. 28: 24, 1966.

443. Stone, H. H., and Fabian, T. C.: Peritoneal dialysis in the treatment of acute alcoholic pancreatitis. Surg. Gynecol. Obstet. 150: 878, 1980.

444. Struve, C.: Sonographische Pankreasdiagnostik. Möglichkeiten und Grenzen. Dtsch. med. Wschr. 106: 67, 1981.

445. Svensson, J.-O.: Role of intravenously infused insulin in treatment of acute pancreatitis. A double-blind study. Scand. J. Gastroent. 10: 487, 1975.

446. Tasman-Jones, C., and Abraham, A.: Hyperlipemia and pancreatitis. Amer. J. Dig. Dis. 18: 767, 1973.

447. Tejerina-Fortheringham, W.: Acute pancreatitis. Pathophysiology and treatment. Gastroenterology 20: 677, 1949.

448. Thal, A., and Brackney, E.: Acute hemorrhagic pancreatic necrosis produced by local Shwartzman reaction. JAMA 155: 569, 1954.

449. Thal, A., Kobold, E. E., and Hollenberg, M. J.: The release of vasoactive substances in acute pancreatitis. Amer. J. Surg. 105: 708, 1963.

450. Theisinger, W., Haas-Denk, S., and Muth, G.: Zur Inhibitor-Therapie bei der Pankreatitis. Med. Welt 28: 1961, 1977.

451. Thiel, A.: Untersuchungen über das Gefässystem des Pankreasläppchens bei verschiedenen Säugern mit besonderer Berücksichtigung der Kapillarknäuel der Langerhansschen Inseln. Z. Zellforsch. 39: 339, 1954.

452. Thomas, J. E.: Neural regulation of pancreatic secretion. In: C. F. Code and W. Heidel (Eds.): Handbook of Physiology, Sect. 6: Alimentary Canal, Vol. II: Secretion. American Physiological Society (Washington, D.C.), 1967.

453. Todd, A.: The histological localization of fibrinolysin activator. J. Path. Bact. 78: 281, 1959.

454. Trapnell, J. E.: The natural history and prognosis of acute pancreatitis. Ann. Royal Coll. Surgeons 38: 265, 1966.

455. Trapnell, J. E.: The pathophysiology of acute pancreatitis and the use of Trasylol in treatment. Acta Anaesthesiol. Belg. 27 (Suppl.): 350, 1976.

456. Trapnell, J. E.: Pathophysiology of acute pancreatitis. World J. Surg. 5: 319, 1981.

457. Trapnell, J. E., and Anderson, M. C.: Role of early laparotomy in acute pancreatitis. Ann. Surg. 165: 49, 1967.

458. Trapnell, J. E., Rigby, C. C., Talbot, C. H., and Duncan, E. H. L.: A controlled trial of Trasylol in the treatment of acute pancreatitis. Brit. J. Surg. 61: 177, 1974.

459. Tuzhilin, S. A., and Dreiling, D. A.: Cardiovascular lesions in pancreatitis. Am. J. Gastroenterol. 63: 381, 1975.

460. Tykkä, H., Mahlberg, H. K., Pantzar, O., and Tallberg, T.: Phospholipase A₂ inhibitors and their possible clinical use in the treatment of acute pancreatitis. Scand. J. Gastroent. 15: 519, 1980.

461. Usadel, K. H., Leuschner, U., and Überla, K. K.: Treatment of acute pancreatitis with somatostatin: A multicenter double-blind trial. New Eng. J. Med. 303: 999, 1980.

462. Usadel, K. H., Schwedes, K., Wdowinski, J., Althoff, P., Seiffert, U. B., Paptis, S., Klempa, I., Strohm, W. D., and Leuschner, U.: Untersuchungen zum kurativen Effekt von Somatostatin bei der akuten Pankreatitis. Verh. Dtsch. Ges. Inn. Med. 85: 591, 1979.

463. Van der Spuy, S.: Endoscopic sphincterotomy in the management of gallstone pancreatitis. Endoscopy 13: 25, 1981.

464. Veghelyi, P. V., Kemeny, T. T., Pozsonyi, J., and Sos, J.: Toxic lesions of the pancreas. Amer. J. Dis. Child. 80: 390, 1950.

465. Autio, V., Juusela, E., and Laushahti, K.: Resection of the pancreas for acute hemorrhagic and necrotizing pancreatitis. World J. Surg. 3: 631, 1979.

466. Vykuril, J.: Pankreasnekrose als Komplikation der Hydrochlorothiazidbehandlung. Cs. Gastroent. Vyz. 20: 136, 1966.

467. Walters, R. L., Gaspard, D. J., and Germann, T. D.: Traumatic pancreatitis. Amer. J. Surg. 111: 364, 1966.

468. Wanke, M.: Isthmusblockade und Hypoxie als Ursachen chronisch rezidivierender wie akuter tryptischer Pankreatitis. Gastroenterologia 103: 103, 1965.

469. Wanke, M.: Lipolytische und proteolytische Form der akuten experimentellen Pankreatitis. Thesis, Heidelberg, 1966.

470. Wanke, M.: Pathologico-anatomical results with acute pancreatitis. In: Recent advances in gastroenterology. Proceedings of the 3rd World Congress of Gastroenterology, Vol. IV, p. 335. Tokyo, 1967.

471. Wanke, M.: Experimentelle Pankreatitis. Proteolytische, lipolytische und biliäre Form. Thieme (Stuttgart), 1968.

472. Wanke, M.: Morphologische Befunde bei der experimentellen akuten Pan-

kreatitis. Gastro-Enterologie (Antwerp) 12: 132, 1969.

473. Wanke, M.: Experimental acute pancreatitis. Current Topics in Pathology, Vol. 52. Springer (Berlin–Heidelberg–New York), 1970.

474. Wanke, M.: Patho- und Morphogenese akuter Pankreatitiden nebst Bemerkungen zur Klinikopathologie. Med. Welt 21: (N.F.): 1226, 1970.

475. Wanke, M.: Die lipolytische Pankreatitis im Kindesalter. Verh. dtsch. Ges. Path. 55: 502, 1971.

476. Wanke, M.: Postoperative Pankreatitis. In: H. Chiari and M. Wanke: Ösophagus, Magen. Spezielle pathologische Anatomie, Vol. II/1, p. 842. Springer (Berlin–Heidelberg–New York), 1971.

477. Wanke, M.: Significance of lipolytic pancreatitis in childhood in the development of acute relapsing pancreatitis. Beitr. Pathol. 146: 272, 1972.

478. Wanke, M.: Akute Pankreaserkrankungen. In: M. M. Forell (Ed.): Handbuch der inneren Medizin, Vol. 3/6, 5th ed. Springer (Berlin–Heidelberg–New York), 1976.

479. Wanke, M.: Gibt es eine urämische Gastritis? Schwerpunkt Med. 3 (4), 1980.

480. Wanke, M.: Morphogenesis of acute pancreatitis. In: Scuro, Dagradi (Eds.): Topics in acute and chronic pancreatitis, p. 93. Springer (Berlin-Heidelberg–New York), 1981.

481. Wanke, M., and Baumann, A.: Pankreaskarzinom: Chronische Pankreatitis – eine Präkanzerose? Diagnostik 13: 278, 1980.

482. Wanke, M., Geiger, V., and Bokelmann, D.: Pathologisch-anatomische Befunde an Leber und Pankreas bei Erkrankungen des Gallengangsystems. Med. Welt 20 (N.F.): 765, 1969.

483. Wanke, M., and Griss, P.: Metastasierendes Nebennierenrindencarcinom mit Cushing-Syndrom und lipolytischer Pankreatitis. Morgagni II, 4: 267, 1969.

484. Wanke, M., and Grözinger, K. H.: Organveränderungen bei experimenteller Pankreatitis. Langenbecks Arch. klin. Chir. 310: 36, 1965.

485. Wanke, M., and Horeyseck, G.: Beziehungen zwischen Nebennierenrinde und lipolytischer Pankreatitis. Demonstriert am Modell der "Cortison-Pankreatitis". Z. Gastroent. 8: 86, 1970.

486. Wanke, M., and Nagel, W.: Degranulierung des exkretorischen Pankreas und autodigestive Pankreatitis.

Verh. dtsch. Ges. Path. 52: 311, 1968.

487. Wanke, M., Nagel, W., Linder, M. M., and Sebening, H.: Über die Stellung der Phospholipase A im Ablauf der akuten Pankreatitis. Z. Gastroent. 6: 434, 1968.

488. Wanke, M., Nagel, W., and Willig, F.: Formen der experimentellen Pankreatitis pathoanatomisch gesehen. Frankf. Z. Path. 75: 207, 1966.

489. Wanke, M., Pfriender, H., Frank, P., Grözinger, K. H., and Bokelmann, D.: Beziehungen zwischen morphologischen und hämodynamischen Veränderungen im postpankreatitischen Schock und ihre therapeutische Beeinflussung. Med. Welt 21 (N.F.): 1238, 1970.

490. Wanke, M., Schmidt, J., and Höhn, N.: Nierenschädigung im postpankreatischen Schock und ihre therapeutische Beeinflussung. Experimentelle und kliniko-pathoanatomische Befunde. In: Neue Aspekte der Trasylol-Therapie 5, p. 83. Schattauer (Stuttgart–New York), 1972.

491. Wanke, M., and Schumann, G.: Pathoanatomisches Bild des Schocks und seiner verschiedenen Formen. Chirurg 45: 97, 1974.

492. Wanke, M., Wegener, K., and Lahmann, H.: Einbaurate von Enzymeiweissraten in das Rattenpankreas nach Adrenalektomie unter Cortison. Virchows Arch. Abt. A, 350: 275, 1970.

493. Warshaw, A. L. O., and Hara, P. J.: Susceptibility of the pancreas to ischemic injury in shock. Ann. Surg. 188: 197, 1978.

494. Warshaw, A. L., Imbembo, A. L., Civetta, J. M., and Daggett, W. M.: Surgical intervention in acute necrotizing pancreatitis. Amer. J. Surg. 127: 484, 1974.

495. Warshaw, A. L., and Lee, K.-H.: The mechanism of increased renal clearance of amylase in acute pancreatitis. Gastroenterology 71: 388, 1976.

496. Waterman, N. G., Walsky, R., Kasdan, M. L., and Abrams, B. L.: The treatment of acute hemorrhagic pancreatitis by sump drainage. Surg. Gynecol. Obstet. 126: 963, 1968.

497. Watts, J. T.: Total pancreatectomy for fulminant pancreatitis. Lancet II: 384, 1963.

498. Webster, M. E., and Clark, W. R.: Significance of kallikrein-kallidinogen-kallidin system in shock. Am. J. Physiol. 197: 406, 1959.

499. Weiner, H. A., and Tennant, R.: A statistical study of acute hemorrhagic pancreatitis (hemorrhagic necrosis of pan-

creas). Amer. J. Med. Sci. 196: 167, 1938.

500. Weiss, H., Weiss, A., Keller, W., Rethel, R., and Ranft, K.: Der Stellenwert der Sonographie in der Diagnostik und Therapie der akuten Pankreatitis. Intensivmedizin 17: 80, 1980.

501. Wenz, W.: Abdominale Angiographie. Angiographische Befunde bei der Pankreatitis. Springer (Berlin–Heidelberg–New York), 1972.

502. Werle, E., and Berck, U.: Zur Kenntnis des Kallikreins. Angew. Chem. 60: 53, 1948.

503. White, T. T.: Acute pancreatitis. In: H. F. Conn (Ed.): Current Therapy 1974. Saunders (London–Toronto), 1974.

504. White, T. T., and Heimbach, D. M.: Sequestrectomy and hyperalimentation in the treatment of hemorrhagic pancreatitis. Amer. J. Surg. 132: 270, 1976.

505. Wilkinson, M. L., O'Driscoll, R., and Kiernan, T. J.: Cimetidine and pancreatitis. Lancet I: 610, 1981.

506. Williams Russel, A., Caldwell, B. F., and Wilson, S. E.: Idiopathic hereditary pancreatitis. Arch. Surg. 117: 408, 1982.

507. Wilson, C. D., Breckenridge, W. C., and Little, J. A.: Inheritance of a lipoprotein C II deficiency with hypertriglyceridemia and pancreatitis. New Eng. J. Med. 26: 1421, 1978.

508. Witte, S.: Bluterkrankungen und Pankreas. In: M. M. Forell (Ed.): Handbuch der inneren Medizin, 5th ed., Vol. 3/6. Springer (Berlin–Heidelberg–New York), 1976.

509. Zayadin, K., and Kirsch, K.: Ergebnisse der Behandlung der akuten Pankreatitis mit und ohne Kalzitonin. Zbl. Chir. 106: 161, 1981.

510. Zick, R., Meyer, Th., and Freise, J.: Hyperosmolares Koma bei Pankreatitis unter Somatostatinbehandlung. Dtsch. med. Wschr. 106: 963, 1981.

Subject Index